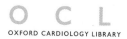

OXFORD CARDIOLOGY LIBRARY

Cardioprotection

Foreword

Coronary heart disease remains the world's biggest killer causing in excess of seven million deaths each year. In recent years, particularly in richer nations, systematic implementation of health policies in the areas of prevention and treatment have led to substantial falls in mortality from cardiac disease but it remains the biggest killer. In developing nations, the epidemic seems to be gathering pace at an alarming rate. So we cannot be complacent in our search for optimal interventions across the whole course of an individual's lifespan whether that relates to life-style, metabolic status, cardiovascular risk, acute episodes of cardiac disease or cardiac procedures in the catheter laboratory and the operating room.

This short text brings together the world's leading experts across all these domains exploring the pathophysiology of myocardial ischaemia and reperfusion, how the myocardium suffers damage, how it might be protected by 'conditioning', how risk factors can be modified and how the risk of damage can be ameliorated during acute cardiac episodes and cardiac procedures. Importantly, this handbook brings together the very latest knowledge and understanding that reflects the varied expertise of the authors, ranging as it does from the laboratory and basic science through practical approaches in primary care to the emergency room, the cardiac care unit, the catheter laboratory and the operating theatre. This text rehearses the many and varied opportunities for intervening to improve outcomes utilising the latest understanding of the mechanisms of coronary heart disease at its various stages.

The range of topics covered is extensive and will surely be of interest to a wide range of clinicians and scientists working in the field. There cannot be many volumes that cover cardioprotection from so many angles while exploring such varied topics as prevention, fibrinolysis, primary coronary angioplasty, stem cells, the many pharmacological interventions as well as the novel and emerging cardioprotective strategies.

Professor Roger Boyle CBE,
National Director for Heart Disease and Stroke,
Department of Health,
United Kingdom.

Symbols and abbreviations

ACE	angiotensin converting enzyme
ACS	Acute coronary syndromes
AMI	acute myocardial infarction
ARB	angiotensin receptor blocker
ATP	adenosine triphosphate
BARI	Bypass Angioplasty Revascularization Investigation Myocardial Jeopardy Index Myocardial Jeopardy Index
CABG	coronary artery bypass graft
CCU	Coronary Care Unit
CHD	Coronary heart disease
DIGAMI	Diabetes Mellitus Insulin—Glucose Infusion in Acute Myocardial Infarction
ECG	electrocardiogram
ERK	extracellular signal-related kinase
FRISC	Fragmin during Instability in Coronary Artery Disease
GIK	glucose-insulin-potassium
ICU	Medical Intensive Care Unit
IPC	ischaemic preconditioning
LV	left ventricular
MARIA	Melatonin Adjunct in the acute myocardial Infarction treated with Angioplasty
MIDCAB	minimally invasive direct coronary artery bypass
mPTP	mitochondrial permeability transition pore
MRI	magnetic resonance imaging
MSC	mesenchymal stem cells
MVO	microvascular obstruction
NHE	sarcolemmal Na^+-H^+ exchanger
NSTEMI	non-ST elevation myocardial infarction
OPCAB	off-pump coronary artery bypass
PKC	protein kinase C

PMI	perioperative myocardial infarction
PPCI	primary percutaneous coronary intervention
PTCA	percutaneous coronary intervention
RAS	renin-angiotensin system
RAAS	renin-angiotensin-aldosterone system
RIPC	remote ischaemic preconditioning
RIPost	remote ischaemic postconditioning
RISK	Reperfusion Injury Salvage Kinase
SPECT	single photon emission computed tomography
STEMI	ST-elevation myocardial infarction
SWOP	second window of preconditioning
TIMI	Thrombolysis in Myocardial Infarction
UFH	unfractioned heparin

Contributors

Dr Michael Cohen
Department of Physiology,
College of Medicine, University
of South Alabama, Alabama, USA.
*Chapter 8 Endogenous
Mechanisms of Cardioprotection*

Dr Dana Dawson
Centre for Cardiovascular Science,
Edinburgh University,
Edinburgh, UK.
*Chapter 4 Anti-Platelet
and Anti-Thrombotic Therapy
Post-AMI*

Prof. James Downey
Department of Physiology,
College of Medicine,
University of South Alabama,
Alabama, USA.
*Chapter 8 Endogenous
Mechanisms of Cardioprotection*

Prof. Keith Fox
Centre for Cardiovascular Science,
Edinburgh University,
Edinburgh, UK.
*Chapter 4 Anti-Platelet and
Anti-Thrombotic Therapy Post-AMI*

Dr Derek J. Hausenloy
The Hatter Cardiovascular Institute,
University College London,
London, UK.
*Chapter 1 An Introduction to
Cardioprotection
Chapter 5 Coronary No-Reflow and
(Microvascular Obstruction)
Chapter 11 Novel
Cardioprotective Strategies*

Prof. Richard Hobbs
The Department of Primary
Care and General Practice,
The University of Birmingham,
Birmingham, UK.
*Chapter 2 Primary Prevention
of Coronary Heart Disease*

Prof. Robert A. Kloner
Heart Institute, Good
Samaritan Hospital,
University of Southern
California, Los Angeles, USA.
*Chapter 9 Adjunctive
Reperfusion Therapy Post-AMI*

Prof. Philippe Menasché
Hôpital Européen Georges
Pompidou and Paris-Descartes
University, Department of
Cardiovascular Surgery and
INSERM U633, Paris, France.
*Chapter 10 Stem Cell Therapy
Post-AMI*

Prof. Lionel Opie
The Hatter Institute for
Cardiovascular Research,
University of Cape Town,
Cape Town, South Africa.
*Chapter 6 Optimal Medical
Therapy Post-AMI*

Prof. John Pepper
National Heart and Lung
Institute,
The Royal Brompton Hospital,
London, UK.
*Chapter 7 Cardioprotection
During Cardiac Surgery*

Dr Thorsten Reffelmann
Heart Institute,
Good Samaritan Hospital,
University of Southern
California, Los Angeles, USA.
*Chapter 9 Adjunctive
Reperfusion Therapy
Post-AMI*

Prof. Maarten Simoons
Thoraxcenter, Erasmus
Medical Center,
Rotterdam, The Netherlands.
*Chapter 3 Percutaneous
Coronary Intervention and
Thrombolysis in AMI and
other ACS*

Dr Frans Visser
Thoraxcenter, Erasmus
Medical Center,
Rotterdam, The Netherlands.
*Chapter 3 Percutaneous Coronary
Intervention and Thrombolysis in
AMI and other ACS*

Prof. Derek Yellon
The Hatter Cardiovascular
Institute, University College
London, London, UK.
*Chapter 1 An Introduction to
Cardioprotection
Chapter 5 Coronary No-Reflow
and Microvascular Obstruction
Chapter 11 Novel
Cardioprotective Strategies*

Chapter 1

An Introduction to Cardioprotection

Derek Hausenloy & Derek Yellon

Key points

- In its broadest sense, the term 'cardioprotection' encompasses 'all mechanisms and means that contribute to the preservation of the heart by reducing or even preventing myocardial damage'
- However, for the purposes of this book, the term 'cardioprotection' will refer to the endogenous mechanisms and therapeutic strategies that reduce or prevent myocardial damage induced by acute ischaemia-reperfusion injury
- In this context, cardioprotection begins with the primary prevention of coronary heart disease and includes the reduction of myocardial injury sustained during coronary artery bypass graft surgery, and an acute myocardial infarction, conditions with considerable morbidity and mortality
- An understanding of the pathophysiology of acute myocardial ischaemia-reperfusion injury is essential when designing new cardioprotective strategies
- Several methods exist for both quantifying myocardial damage induced by acute ischaemia-reperfusion injury and for assessing myocardial salvage following the application of cardioprotective strategies
- Importantly, novel cardioprotective strategies must be capable of preventing and reducing myocardial damage over and above that provided by current optimal therapy.

1.1 A brief history of cardioprotection

One definition for cardioprotection includes 'all mechanisms and means that contribute to the preservation of the heart by reducing or even preventing myocardial damage' (Kubler & Haas, 1996). However, this broad term does not specify the pathophysiological process by which the myocardial injury is incurred. For the purposes of this book, we will be focusing on acute ischaemia-reperfusion injury as the major determinant of myocardial damage, and therefore in this context, the term 'cardioprotection' will refer to the endogenous mechanisms and therapeutic strategies that reduce or prevent myocardial damage incurred as a consequence of acute ischaemia-reperfusion injury.

It is generally agreed that the research field of cardioprotection was born over 35 years ago in the early 1970's in seminal experimental studies led by Eugene Braunwald's group (Maroko et al.,1971), with the discovery that myocardial damage sustained during coronary artery occlusion could be limited by pharmacological agents or interventional strategies which reduced myocardial oxygen consumption or enhanced myocardial anaerobic metabolism. Subsequent pioneering experimental studies first demonstrated that restoring coronary blood flow, following a three hour occlusion, dramatically reduced myocardial infarct size in canine hearts (Ginks et al., 1972), giving rise to the current clinical practice of using thrombolytic therapy and primary percutaneous coronary intervention to establish coronary artery blood flow following an acute myocardial infarction. Until this day, early and complete myocardial reperfusion remains the most powerful intervention for reducing myocardial infarct size. However, despite optimal therapy the morbidity and mortality of an acute myocardial infarction remains significant, necessitating the development of new treatment strategies for protecting the heart against myocardial ischaemia-reperfusion injury. The development of novel cardioprotective strategies requires an understanding of the metabolic and biochemical events occurring during acute myocardial ischaemia-reperfusion injury.

1.2 Pathophysiology of acute myocardial ischaemia-reperfusion injury

An acute myocardial infarction is heralded by the rupture of an unstable coronary atherosclerotic plaque and the subsequent thrombus formation which completely occludes blood flow in the epicardial coronary artery, rendering the myocardium supplied by the infarct-related coronary artery acutely ischaemic. Experimental studies using canine hearts have reported that prolonged myocardial ischaemia induces cardiomyocyte necrosis beginning in the subendocardium after 40 minutes of ischaemia, which progresses like a 'wave-front' to the epicardium resulting in a transmural myocardial infarct (Reimer et al., 1977).

During myocardial ischaemia, cardiomyocytes generate lactic acid from anaerobic metabolism, which reduces intracellular pH, activating the sarcolemmal Na^+-H^+ exchanger which allows the cell to extrude H^+ ions at the expense of intracellular Na^+ accumulation. The rise in intracellular Na^+ activates the Na^+-Ca^{2+} exchanger which rids the cell of Na^+ in exchange for Ca^{2+} resulting in the intracellular accumulation of the latter, and the subsequent Ca^{2+} loading of mitochondria. Meanwhile, in an attempt to maintain the electrochemical gradient required to drive mitochondrial oxidative phosphorylation, available reserves of ATP are broken down to ADP and phosphate resulting in further ATP depletion and high mitochondrial levels of phosphate.

After a prolonged period of myocardial ischaemia, the cardiomyocyte is acidic (pH <7.0), overloaded with calcium and phosphate, and depleted of ATP (this is depicted in Figure 1.1). Restoring coronary blood flow to the ischaemic myocardium results in a further metabolic and biochemical insult to the vulnerable myocardium in the first few minutes of reperfusion. The presence of oxygen allows the re-energisation of mitochondria generating a burst of detrimental oxidative stress in the first few minutes of myocardial reperfusion. Mitochondrial re-energisation restores the electrochemical gradient which allows a rapid influx of calcium into mitochondria. The reperfusion of ischaemic myocardium washes out the lactic acid which together with the actions of the Na^+-H^+ exchanger and the Na^+-HCO-symporter, rapidly restores intracellular pH to the physiological range. All these factors act in concert to induce cardiomyocyte death by two related mechanisms: (a) promoting the opening of the mitochondrial permeability transition pore (mPTP), a non-selective high-conductance inner mitochondrial membrane channel which uncouples oxidative phosphorylation and induces mitochondrial swelling and rupture (Hausenloy & Yellon, 2003); and (b) cardiomyocyte hypercontracture.

Experimental studies have clearly demonstrated that individually targeting mediators of lethal reperfusion injury can reduce myocardial infarct size by nearly half, suggesting that lethal reperfusion injury contributes 25–50% of the final myocardial infarct size (Yellon & Hausenloy, 2007). In this regard, the treatment intervention needs to be applied before or at the immediate onset of myocardial reperfusion to confer cardioprotection (see Figure 1.1).

1.3 Cardioprotection during an AMI

Every year in the US there are 500,000 ST-elevation myocardial infarctions (Antman et al., 2004). In the year 2005, there were 227,000 myocardial infarctions in the UK (http://www.heartstats.org/). Restoring coronary artery flow in the infarct-related artery as soon as possible is the main treatment objective in patients presenting with an acute myocardial infarction (AMI) in order to maximize myocardial

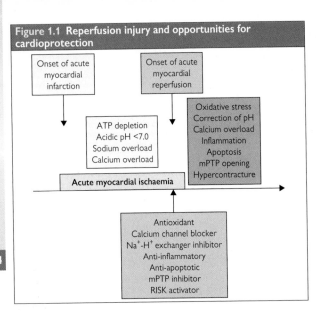

Figure 1.1 Reperfusion injury and opportunities for cardioprotection

Onset of acute myocardial infarction

Onset of acute myocardial reperfusion

ATP depletion
Acidic pH <7.0
Sodium overload
Calcium overload

Oxidative stress
Correction of pH
Calcium overload
Inflammation
Apoptosis
mPTP opening
Hypercontracture

Acute myocardial ischaemia

Antioxidant
Calcium channel blocker
Na⁺-H⁺ exchanger inhibitor
Anti-inflammatory
Anti-apoptotic
mPTP inhibitor
RISK activator

salvage and limit infarct size. This is achieved by thrombolytic therapy or primary percutaneous coronary intervention, depending on the available facilities, the time to presentation and other factors. However, the process of reperfusion itself is capable of exacerbating myocardial injury, thereby mitigating the beneficial effects of timely reperfusion in terms of infarct-size reduction- a phenomenon termed 'lethal reperfusion injury' (Yellon & Hausenloy, 2007). This form of irreversible reperfusion injury is distinct from the reversible forms of myocardial reperfusion injury such as reperfusion arrhythmias and myocardial stunning which are easily dealt with.

However, despite optimal therapy the mortality following an ST-elevation myocardial infarction (STEMI) remains significant at around 10% at one year (Keely et al., 2003). Therefore, to improve clinical outcomes in this patient group, new treatment strategies are required to:

1. reduce the time from symptom onset to an open artery;
2. delay the ischemic myocardial damage occurring prior to myocardial reperfusion;
3. optimise the actual coronary reperfusion procedure;
4. maintain the patency of the infarct-related coronary artery using antiplatelet and antithrombotic therapy;

5. prevent and treat coronary 'no-reflow' thereby maximizing myocardial perfusion;

6. provide reperfusion adjunctive therapy which can prevent and reduce 'lethal reperfusion injury'.

1.4 **Cardioprotection during CABG surgery**

Every year in the US there are about 200,000 CABG operations. In the UK, nearly 29,000 patients have CABG surgery every year (www.heartstats.org). For patients undergoing planned low-risk surgery the mortality is about 2–3%. However, given the recent advances in PCI, the aging population, the prevalence of co-morbidities such as diabetes and obesity, increasingly higher-risk and more complicated patients are being operated on resulting in mortality rates of up to 20%. Furthermore, about 20% of patients undergoing CABG surgery experience a perioperative myocardial infarction (PMI), which is associated with worse clinical outcomes. Even in the absence of a PMI, significant myocardial damage can occur during surgery in response to acute myocardial ischaemia-reperfusion injury, direct myocardial handling and coronary embolisation, resulting in poorer clinical outcomes. Therefore, to improve clinical outcomes in this patient group, new treatment strategies are required to prevent a PMI or reduce the damage sustained by the myocardium if a PMI does occur. In addition, cardioprotective strategies need to be developed to minimize the myocardial damage which occurs during cardiac surgery.

Clearly, other clinical settings in which acute myocardial ischaemia-reperfusion injury occurs such as in the patients surviving a cardiac arrest, the patients undergoing high-risk elective PCI and in cardiac transplant surgery, may also benefit from the development of new cardioprotective strategies.

1.5 **Quantifying myocardial salvage**

A pre-requisite for assessing the efficacy of a cardioprotection intervention in the setting of CABG surgery and an acute myocardial infarction (AMI) is being able to quantify the extent of myocardial damage. Conversely, the ability to measure myocardial salvage (defined as the potential infarct size minus the actual infarct size) is used to assess the efficacy of treatment strategies aimed at reducing myocardial injury in AMI patients undergoing reperfusion.

About 20% of patients undergoing CABG surgery experience a perioperative myocardial infarction (most often due to acute graft occlusion), defined by a rise of 5x the normal range of serum cardiac enzymes along with relevant ECG changes (Thygesen *et al.*, 2007). In addition, the heart may experience non-specific myocardial injury resulting in the release of cardiac enzymes in the absence of significant ECG changes. Interestingly, the myocardial necrosis which occurs during CABG surgery can be detected by late gadolinium enhancement cardiac MRI scanning (16). Clinical studies suggest that the release of cardiac enzymes during CABG surgery is associated with worse clinical outcomes (Lehrke *et al.*, 2004; Croal *et al.*, 2006).

For AMI patients undergoing reperfusion therapy, the area under the curve of serum cardiac enzymes may provide some indication as to the size of the myocardial infarct, although more reliable methods for determining infarct size are available including nuclear myocardial scans, and late gadolinium enhancement cardiac MRI, as mentioned above. In addition, patients undergoing percutaneous coronary intervention for stable coronary artery disease or non-ST-elevation MI can also experience a peri-procedural MI, defined by a rise of 3x the normal range of serum cardiac enzymes (Thygesen *et al.*, 2007), providing another clinical setting for new cardioprotective strategies.

Whichever method is used to quantify the size of the myocardial infarct, it is essential to be able to measure the myocardium at risk of infarction, thereby allowing the extent of myocardial salvage to be calculated as an indicator of cardioprotection. An estimate of the myocardium at risk of infarction (the ischaemic risk zone) can be provided by: the extent of ST-elevation present on the initial 12-lead ECG: the number of regional wall motion abnormalities present on LV angiography or transthoracic echocardiography: and coronary angiography using the Bypass Angioplasty Revascularization Investigation Myocardial Jeopardy Index Myocardial Jeopardy Index (BARI) and the Alberta Provincial Project for Outcome Assessment in Coronary Heart Disease (APPROACH) scores (Ortiz-Perez *et al.*, 2007). However, a more accurate quantification has conventionally been provided by technetium 99m sestamibi single photon emission computed tomography (SPECT) imaging (Milavetz *et al.*, 1998; Ndrepepa *et al.*, 2004). An injection of the radioisotope technetium immediately prior to myocardial reperfusion delineates the ischaemic risk zone as the area with absent radioisotope uptake. Because of the properties of the radioisotope myocardial perfusion imaging can take place 6–8 hours following the injection. One week later, a further SPECT scan is undertaken which then delineates the myocardial infarct. However, this imaging technique requires the availability of the radioactive tracer 24 hours a day, exposes the patient to a significant radiation dose, lacks resolution and may miss subendocardial myocardial infarcts.

Recent experimental studies suggest that cardiac MRI may also allow quantification of the ischaemic risk zone. It is well-established that delayed gadolinium-enhanced cardiac MRI can demarcate the myocardial infarct in AMI patients undergoing myocardial reperfusion.

Figure 1.2 Imaging the myocardium at risk of infarction in AMI patients

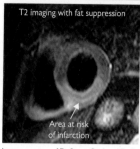

T2 imaging with fat suppression

Area at risk
of infarction

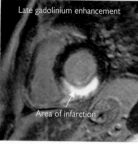

Late gadolinium enhancement

Area of infarction

Images courtesy of Dr Stuart Cook and Dr Declan O'Regan

The ischaemic risk zone has been retrospectively imaged using T2 weighted cardiac MRI scans which detect increased signal intensity due to myocardial oedema which persists for several days following an AMI. Aletras et al., (2006) have demonstrated that T2-weighted myocardial oedema imaging 2 days following an experimental coronary occlusion in canine hearts can accurately depict the ischaemic risk zone. A subsequent study has successfully reported increased myocardial salvage using intravenous beta-blockers in porcine hearts subjected to acute coronary occlusion using this imaging technique (Ibanez et al., 2007). Validation studies in AMI patients are currently underway using modifications of this T2-weighted sequence to determine whether this imaging technique can be applied in the clinical setting (Aletras et al., 2008) (see Figure 1.2).

1.6 Conclusions

Despite current optimal therapy, the morbidity and mortality from coronary heart disease remains significant. Its major clinical manifestations which form the main subjects of this book are the emergent setting of an acute myocardial infarction and the elective setting of coronary artery bypass graft (CABG) surgery. In this context, cardioprotection refers to the endogenous mechanisms and therapeutic strategies that reduce or prevent myocardial damage incurred by acute ischaemia-reperfusion injury in these clinical settings. The development of effective treatment cardioprotective strategies requires a thorough understanding of the underlying pathophysiology of acute myocardial ischaemia-reperfusion injury. This book begins with the primary prevention of coronary heart disease and then reviews the current treatment strategies for reducing myocardial injury in patients presenting with an AMI and in those undergoing CABG surgery. Finally, novel cardioprotective strategies which are currently in development and are undergoing clinical testing will be introduced as a future approach to improving clinical outcomes in patients with coronary heart disease.

Key references

Aletras, A.H., Kellman, P., Derbyshire, J.A., Arai, A.E. (2008). ACUT(2)E TSE-SSFP: A hybrid method for T2-weighted imaging of edema in the heart. *Magn Reson Med*, **59**: 229–235.

Aletras, A.H., Tilak, G.S., Natanzon, A., *et al.*, (2006). Retrospective determination of the area at risk for reperfused acute myocardial infarction with T2-weighted cardiac magnetic resonance imaging: histopathological and displacement encoding with stimulated echoes (DENSE) functional validations. *Circulation*, **113**: 1865–1870.

Antman, E.M., Anbe, D.T., Armstrong, P.W., *et al.*, (2004). ACC/AHA guidelines for the management of patients with ST-elevation myocardial infarction–executive summary: a report of the American College of Cardiology/American Heart Association Task Force on Practice Guidelines (Writing Committee to Revise the 1999 Guidelines for the Management of Patients With Acute Myocardial Infarction). *Circulation*, **110**: 588–636.

Croal, B.L., Hillis, G.S., Gibson, P.H., *et al.*, (2006). Relationship between postoperative cardiac troponin I levels and outcome of cardiac surgery. *Circulation*, **114**: 1468–1475.

Ginks, W.R., Sybers, H.D., Maroko, P.R., *et al.*, (1972). Coronary artery reperfusion. II. Reduction of myocardial infarct size at 1 week after the coronary occlusion. *J Clin Invest*, **51**: 2717–2723.

Hausenloy, D.J., Yellon, D.M. (2003). The mitochondrial permeability transition pore: its fundamental role in mediating cell death during ischaemia and reperfusion. *J Mol Cell Cardiol*, **35**: 339–341.

Ibanez, B., Prat-Gonzalez, S., Speidl, W.S., *et al.*, (2007). Early metoprolol administration before coronary reperfusion results in increased myocardial salvage: analysis of ischemic myocardium at risk using cardiac magnetic resonance. *Circulation*, **115**: 2909–2916.

Keeley, E.C., Boura, J.A., Grines, C.L. (2003). Primary angioplasty versus intravenous thrombolytic therapy for acute myocardial infarction: a quantitative review of 23 randomized trials. *Lancet*, **361**: 13–20.

Kubler, W., Haass, M. (1996). Cardioprotection: definition, classification, and fundamental principles. *Heart*, **75**: 330–333.

Lehrke, S., Steen, H., Sievers, H.H., *et al.*, (2004). Cardiac troponin T for prediction of short- and long-term morbidity and mortality after elective open heart surgery. *Clin Chem* **50**: 1560–1567.

Maroko, P.R., Kjekshus, J.K., Sobel, B.E., *et al.*, (1971). Factors influencing infarct size following experimental coronary artery occlusions. *Circulation*, **43**: 67–82.

Milavetz, J.J., Giebel, D.W., Christian, T.F., et al., (1998). Time to therapy and salvage in myocardial infarction. *J Am Coll Cardiol* **31**: 1246–1251.

Ndrepepa, G., Mehilli, J., Schwaiger, M., et al., (2004). Prognostic value of myocardial salvage achieved by reperfusion therapy in patients with acute myocardial infarction. *J Nucl Med*, **45**: 725–729.

Ortiz-Perez, J.T., Meyers, S.N., Lee, D.C., et al., (2007). Angiographic estimates of myocardium at risk during acute myocardial infarction: validation study using cardiac magnetic resonance imaging. *Eur Heart J* **28**: 1750–1758.

Reimer, K.A., Lowe, J.E., Rasmussen, M.M., Jennings R.B. (1977). The wave-front phenomenon of ischemic cell death. 1. Myocardial infarct size vs duration of coronary occlusion in dogs. *Circulation*, **56**: 786–794.

Selvanayagam, J.B., Searle, N., Neubauer, S., Taggart, D.P. (2006). Correlation of coronary artery bypass surgery-related myonecrosis with grafted vessel calibre: insights from cardiovascular magnetic resonance imaging. *Heart*, **92**: 1329–1330.

Thygesen, K., Alpert, J.S., White, H.D., et al., (2007). Universal definition of myocardial infarction. *Circulation*, **116**: 2634–2653.

Yellon, D.M., Hausenloy, D.J. (2007). Myocardial reperfusion injury. *N Engl J Med*, **357**: 1121–1135.

Chapter 2

Primary Prevention of Coronary Heart Disease

Richard Hobbs

Key points

- Coronary heart disease (CHD) is the leading cause of death and disability in the world
- The evidence base for the causes of CHD and for the interventions which reduce CHD risk is huge
- Since CHD is multi-factorial, risk factors tend to co-exist in many patients, and are multiplicative in their influence on overall risk, making identifying people at highest risk clinically difficult
- CHD risk scores have been developed, based on observed CHD rates amongst well-phenotyped patient cohorts followed up over years. These express absolute risk over a defined period and are the most practical method for determining which people have the most to gain from treatment interventions
- Evidence-based interventions include smoking cessation, lifestyle modification in terms of diet and exercise, anti-hypertensives for elevated blood pressure, and 'statins' for hyperlipidaemia
- Clinical guidelines for CHD prevention provide recommendations on specific targets for blood pressure and lipid-lowering therapy.

2.1 Introduction

The prevention of coronary heart disease (CHD) and the management of established disease remain a key priority for all health systems in order that the onset of secondary complications are delayed or avoided. Coronary heart disease is the leading cause of death and disability in the world (Figure 2.1). Long-term follow-up of patients with CHD have provided an evidence base upon which health professionals can base their interventions to modify CHD risk. Primary

Figure 2.1 Ten leading causes of death and disability in the world

Global leading causes of death and disability
(disability adjusted life years)

	1990			2020	
Rank	Cause	%	Rank	Cause	%
1	Lower respiratory infections	8.2	1	Ischaemic heart disease	5.9
2	Diarrhoeal diseases	7.2	2	Major depression	5.7
3	Perinatal conditions	6.7	3	Road traffic accidents	5.1
4	Major depression	3.7	4	Cerebrovascular disease	4.4
5	Ischaemic heart disease	3.4	5	COPD	4.2
6	Cerebrovascular disease	2.8	6	Lower respiratory infections	3.1
7	Tuberculosis	2.8	7	Tuberculosis	3.0
8	Measles	2.7	8	War	3.0
9	Road traffic accidents	2.5	9	Diarrhoeal diseases	2.7
10	Congenital abnormalities	2.4	10	HIV	2.6

Murray C.J.L. & Lopez, A.D. (eds.) The global burden of disease. The global burden of disease and injury series, Volume 1: a comprehensive assessment of mortality and disability from diseases, injuries, and risk factors in 1990 and projected to 2020, Harvard University Press, Cambridge (1996).

prevention of CHD is important because in at least 50% of cases, it will manifest as an acute myocardial infarction (AMI) or sudden cardiac death. Delaying interventions until people actually present with symptomatic disease, such as angina and an AMI, therefore renders them eligible for secondary prevention, and is therefore not a sensible policy. However, in reference to the primary prevention of CHD, while there is considerable evidence on what to do, in terms of which risk factors are important and how to reduce the impact of these risk factors, data are limited on how this evidence-base should be implemented in clinical practice. One major problem area is how to effectively structure care to identify those individuals who are at greatest risk. Having decided who to treat, current targets for therapy are explicit and achievable for both hypertension and hyperlipidaemia. It is important to appreciate that effective treatment is likely to require multiple drug therapy.

2.2 Major risk factors for CHD

Major non-modifiable risk factors include family history of premature coronary heart disease (CHD), age, gender and ethnicity. Modifiable risk factors include dyslipidaemia (high levels of low-density lipoprotein cholesterol [LDL-C] and triglycerides [TG], and low levels of high-density lipoprotein cholesterol [HDL-C]), hypertension (especially systolic elevation), cigarette smoking and diabetes (MRFIT, 1982; Anderson *et al.*, 1987; Vershuren *et al.*, 1995; MacMahon *et al.*, 1990) (Figure 2.2). One of the most important messages to emerge during

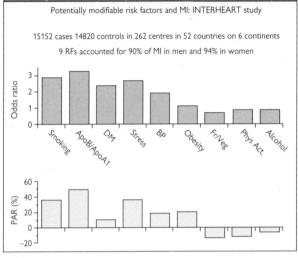

Figure 2.2 Main risk factors associated with coronary heart disease (Yusef et al., 2004)

Potentially modifiable risk factors and MI: INTERHEART study

15152 cases 14820 controls in 262 centres in 52 countries on 6 continents

9 RFs accounted for 90% of MI in men and 94% in women

the past decade is that these risks factors are multiplicative. This has led to the development of algorithm-based risk calculators for predicting an individual's cardiovascular risk over a defined time period.

Studies have shown that 80–90% of CHD patients have at least one of these four modifiable risk factors (MRFIT, 1982; Anderson et al., 1987; Vershuren et al., 1995; MacMahon et al., 1990; Greenland et al., 2003; Khot et al., 2003) and each of these risk factors has a continuous, dose-dependent impact on CHD risk. In addition, treatment of these and other risk factors (e.g. obesity) has been convincingly shown to reduce the risk of CHD events and stroke (Greenland et al., 2003; Khot et al., 2003; Collins et al., 1990; Heart Protection Study 2002; UKPDS 1998). Patients with type 2 diabetes are also at particularly high CHD risk (Haffner et al., 1998), which has resulted in many health systems viewing diabetes as a CHD risk factor equivalent. However, a more accurate interpretation is that diabetes should only represent a CHF risk factor equivalent in people who have had diabetes for some time (this includes those with established diabetes and for those in whom there has been a delay in diagnosis) and in those with multiple risk factors in addition to their diabetes. If diabetes is diagnosed earlier, then the disease confers an intermediate level of risk, higher than the non-diabetic population but lower than those who have suffered actual CHD events. Diabetes is becoming much more common (Mokdad et al., 2000), and secondary risks are therefore a major issue. This is reflected in the National Service Framework (NSF) for diabetes recommendation to intervene earlier with a 'statin' at a 15% 10-year CHD risk rather than a 30% 10-year CHD risk. However, since most guidelines recommend that diabetes is treated as a secondary prevention population, they will not be considered further in this chapter.

It has been known for over 30 years that interventions are needed to treat hypertension and for 15 years to treat hyperlipidaemia. A follow up meta-analysis in 1990 of hypertension intervention trials showed a 42% risk reduction in stroke by treating hypertension and a 14% reduction in CHD (Greenland *et al.*, 2003). Following the earlier clinical trials it was thought that treating hypertension would only influence stroke; however, by pooling the data, treatment was shown to also influence CHD. An interesting observation from the meta-analyses was that while the expected reductions (extrapolated from earlier epidemiological associations) were seen in stroke risk, the blood pressure lowering trials under-performed in observed reductions in CHD compared to the anticipated 20–25% reduction that epidemiological studies had suggested. One explanation for this observation may be that stroke is more closely related to the 'pressor' effect of blood pressure while CHD is more dependent on multifactorial risk. As such, the expected reductions in CHD events were not observed in clinical trials, until attention was directed to reducing lipids.

2.3 Identifying individuals with raised CHD risk

The scale of the task in delivering primary prevention in many healthcare systems is enormous. It is difficult to estimate the level of success being achieved in primary prevention because there exists little reliable data on the denominator at-risk population. However, for example in the UK, the Health Survey for England (Primatesta *et al.*, 2001) gives some indication of the number of people who might be eligible for primary prevention of CHD. In the 1998 survey, more than 25% of the adult population in England had their total cholesterol to HDL-C ratio above 5. Therefore, by using a level of 30% 10-year CHD risk as a treatment threshold, then around 15% of the adult population in the UK would be eligible for intervention. However, using an intervention threshold of 20% 10-year CHD would equate to over 20% of adults being eligible for intervention.

Formal population screening is therefore advocated in the US NCEP ATP III guidelines, which recommend screening for elevated blood pressure and lipids in all adults without CHD every 5 years and in those with CHD every 2–3 years, although there are no data on the cost-effectiveness of this strategy (NCEP ATP III guidelines

2001). A less ambitious alternative would be case-finding those at higher overall CHD risk through formal CHD risk estimation in those patients which have a single CHD risk factor. The European (De Backer et al., 2003) and UK (Joint British Societies, 2005) guidelines advocate such screening in all patients with any individual CHD risk factor, and emphasise the importance of screening close relatives of patients with premature CHD (defined as men <55 years, women <65 years) and persons who belong to families with familial hypercholesterolaemia or other inherited dyslipidaemias.

Coronary heart disease risk estimation can be made using any of the CHD risk calculator tools that are based on observational outcome data from large population cohorts such as the Framingham equation in the US, SCORE in Europe, and UKPDS for those with diabetes. In all CHD risk scores, treatment decisions are based on the likelihood that an individual will have an event over a given period of time (the absolute CHD risk). This replaces decision-making based on individual risk factor level, as it is now recognised that a patient with borderline elevations in multiple risk factors may be at greater risk of a major coronary event or stroke than a patient with a single established CHD risk factor. To facilitate the assessment of these risk factors, algorithms have been incorporated into clinical guidelines. The algorithms assign points to a patient according to their risk factor exposure. The sum of these points is then used to calculate a patient's total 10-year risk of CHD (NCEP ATP III guidelines) (NCEP ATP III guidelines 2001) or cardiovascular death (Third Joint European guidelines) (De Backer et al., 2003) (see Tables 2.1 and 2.2).

None of the CHD risk scores are perfect (explaining the proliferation of a variety of methods) and they cannot be applied to a broad patient population. For example, the Framingham data probably over-estimates risks in modern populations (because the background risk of CHD has declined in many countries), especially in Southern Europe. Also, the SCORE data only estimates cardiovascular deaths rather than all events. However, all CHD risk scores succeed in identifying those patients most at risk allowing efficient targeting of evidenced-base therapies. Clinical studies suggest that patients will derive significant vascular gains from treating CHD 10-year risk levels down to 6%, so even if the scores do slightly over-estimate risk, a threshold set at 20% 10 year CHD risk is set way above the levels for which the evidence of benefit is established.

2.4 **Reducing CHD risk in primary prevention**

Using tools such as these CHD risk prediction charts or related computerised algorithms will guide which patients should be targeted

Table 2.1 NCEP ATP III LDL-C treatment goals

Risk category	LDL-C goal mmol/L (mg/dL)	LDL-C level for lifestyle changes mmol/L (mg/dL)	LDL-C level to initiate pharmacotherapy mmol/L (mg/dL)
CHD risk (10-yr CHD risk >20%)	<2.5 (<100) Goal for high risk <1.8 (<70)	≥2.5 (≥100)	≥2.5 (≥100) May consider pharmacotherapy <2.5 (<100)
2+ CHD risk factors (10-yr CHD risk ≤20%)	<3.3 (<130) Optional goal <2.5 (<100)	≥3.3 (≥130)	10-yr risk 10–20%: ≥3.3 (≥130) May consider pharmacotherapy 2.5–3.3 (100–129) 10-yr risk <10%: ≥4.1 (≥160)
0–1 CHD risk factors	<4.1 (<160)	≥4.1 (≥160)	≥4.9 (≥190) May consider pharmacotherapy 4.1–4.8 (160–189)

in terms of primary prevention. Once a decision is made to intervene, all CHD prevention guidelines provide explicit, relatively simple and achievable targets for both hypertension and dyslipidaemia. The first step to reduce CHD risk involves making lifestyle changes. Patients usually require behavioural counselling on appropriate lifestyle changes, including the reduction of body weight, dietary changes, smoking cessation and increased physical exercise. Numerous interventions to assist smoking cessation have been evaluated and physician guidelines published (West *et al.*, 2000). Normalisation of weight, increased consumption of fruit and vegetables, decreased intake of saturated fats (<10% of calories), salt (<6 g/day) and free sugars, and increased activity levels reduces CHD risk. Data suggest that a therapeutic diet can provide moderate reductions in cholesterol levels, and may regress coronary atherosclerosis (Walden *et al.*, 1997; Watts *et al.*, 1992). There is also limited evidence that reducing cholesterol levels with diet alone may contribute to a reduction in coronary events (Arntzenius *et al.*, 1985; Ornish *et al.*, 1990). The lipid profile can also be positively influenced by increased physical activity and weight reduction, with addition of an average of 30 minutes of exercise a day to the diet recommended in the NCEP ATP III guidelines reduced LDL-C levels by 9.3% after 6 weeks (Welty *et al.*, 2002). Exercise and diet can further aid weight reduction, which has a beneficial effect on lipid levels and CVD rates.

Table 2.2 Third Joint European Task Force LDL-C treatment goals

10-yr risk category	LDL-C goal mmol/L (mg/dL)	Initial treatment	Follow up
CHD/ diabetes	<2.5 (<100)	Lifestyle advice; Pharmacotherapy, as appropriate	
≥5%	<3.0 (<115)	Measure fasting total chol, HDL-C* & TG* Lifestyle advice for at least 3 months	Re-measure lipids: a) Total chol <5 mmol/L (190 mg/dL) & LDL-C goal achieved, maintain lifestyle advice & follow up at 1 year. If total risk remains ≥5%, consider pharmacotherapy b) Total chol ≥5 mmol/L (190 mg/dL) & LDL-C goal not achieved, maintain lifestyle advice & initiate pharmacotherapy. If risk remains ≥5%, use pharmacotherapy
<5%	<3.0 (<115)	Lifestyle advice	Follow up at a minimum of 5 year intervals

* No specific treatment goals defined for HDL-C/TG. HDL-C <1.0 mmol/L (40 mg/dL) in men and 1.2 mmol/L (46 mg/dL) in women, and TG >1.7 mmol/L (150 mg/dL) serve as markers of increased risk. HDL-C and TG levels should also be used to guide the choice of pharmacotherapy.

A meta-analysis in 1990 of hypertension intervention trials showed a 42% risk reduction in stroke by treating hypertension and a 14% reduction in coronary heart disease. Results from the Hypertension Optimal Treatment (HOT) trial (Hansson et al., 1998) have provided the main rationale for guideline recommendations on target blood pressure. HOT showed that the risk of a major cardiovascular event was significantly reduced if systolic pressure was reduced to below 150 mmHg, and that optimal systolic blood pressure was 138 mmHg. For diastolic pressure, <90 mmHg was significantly better than 95 mmHg in reducing risk, and the optimal level was 83 mmHg. The HOT trial also demonstrated that targets that are historically considered to be difficult can be achieved in routine primary care practice, provided that combination therapy is used. At the end of the five-year trial, only one-third of patients were taking a single drug. Forty-eight per cent of patients were taking two drugs and 20% were taking three or four drugs.

Trials have also shown that even in high-risk hypertension groups, such as patients with diabetes, an incremental benefit is achieved by more aggressive blood pressure control. In the United Kingdom Prospective Diabetes Study (UKPDS), tight control (144/82 mmHg) was associated with a 24% reduction in risk of cardiovascular events compared with less tight control (154/87 mmHg) (Wilson *et al.*, 1998). However, attention to blood pressure should not be at the exclusion of glycaemic control. In UKPDS, the people who had the best outcomes were those who had the tightest blood pressure control and also the tightest HbA_{1C} control. All risk factors need to be treated equally aggressively.

For lipid lowering, it was estimated from the MRFIT study that every 0.5 mmol/l increase in total cholesterol corresponds to an increase in CVD mortality risk of 12 per cent and an increase in mortality risk of 17 per cent when adjusted for regression dilution bias (MRFIT trial, 1982). This enhanced risk can be modified by cholesterol reduction, with most evidence for statins and reduction of LDL-cholesterol: in a recent meta-analysis of the major statin lipid reduction trials, every 1 mmol/l reduction in TC was associated with a 23% reduction in CHD and 21% risk reduction in all CVD events (Brady & Betteridge, 2003). There is also evidence from intervention trials that benefit of this magnitude is achieved whichever method is used to reduce cholesterol levels. Targets for LDL-C were set initially on the basis of older landmark statin studies (Nissen *et al.*, 2004; Cannon *et al.*, 2004), however some guidelines recommend to further reduce these goals (Grundy *et al.*, 2004) on the basis of more recent trials indicating that risk of cardiovascular disease can be further lowered by treating to more aggressive targets (Nissen *et al.*, 2004; Cannon *et al.*, 2004). Furthermore, mortality improvements have been observed in patients with multiple risk factors, but in only those with normal to mildly elevated cholesterol at baseline (mean total cholesterol ≤6.5 mmol/L in ASCOT study).

2.5 **Public perceptions of CHD risk**

Perhaps, one of the greatest challenges facing clinicians after having identified the patient group at greatest CHD risk, is to maintain patients on the evidence-based interventions which reduce their CHD risk. Many patients discontinue therapy, often within 12 months of starting, particularly those on statin therapy. Part of this poor adherence may be related to perceived risks of CHD within the general population. A survey in five European countries asked a random 5,000 members of the general public for their opinions about CHD risk. Only 45% of people surveyed correctly identified CHD as the leading cause of death in their country (UKPDS, 1998). People mistakenly believed that cancer was a greater personal risk. There were also significant gaps in knowledge about what causes cardiovascular disease. General practitioners in the same countries were also surveyed and 92% of physicians thought that their patients would know that elevated cholesterol was associated with cardiovascular disease (Anderson *et al.*, 2001). In reality, less than half of the public recognised an association between cholesterol and elevated risk; stress was rated as more important than cholesterol. Thirty per cent did not recognise an association between smoking and coronary heart disease and only a quarter were aware of the relevance of the different lipid fractions (UKPDS, 1998). There are therefore important issues to tackle relating to increasing the general public's understanding of cardiovascular disease.

2.6 **Conclusions**

The sheer burden of coronary heart disease legitimises CHD primary prevention as a global priority for health-care services. There is a need to structure care to identify those at risk, and then to apply structured lifestyle and therapeutic interventions and monitoring of these patients. The call-recall systems that are applied so effectively in terms of cancer prevention need to be applied to CHD primary prevention. There should be some optimism that CHD prevention will improve. It is known that offering brief advice and nicotine replacement therapy to smokers, and doing this repeatedly, will achieve success (around 15%) in helping people to stop smoking. Screening and structured follow-up clinics are known to improve care in chronic disorders: for blood pressure there needs to be opportunistic screening, and lipid levels need to be checked in people with hypertension or diabetes, and from the age of 18 in the case of premature cardiovascular disease in a parent (father <55 years, mother <65 years). Checks should also be made for diabetes, based on symptoms and obesity. In addition to the emphasis on these primary cardiovascular risk factors, major problems that need closer attention include the rising incidence of obesity, the metabolic syndrome and diabetes. However, in addition to these physician-led CHD prevention strategies, Government policies on food subsidy and taxation, alcohol licensing, banning smoking where feasible, and access to exercise are just as crucial for improving the nation's cardiovascular health.

Key references

Anderson, J.W., Konz, E.C. (2001). Obesity and disease management: effects of weight loss on co-morbid conditions. *Obes Res*, **9** Suppl 4: 326S–334S.

Anderson, K.M., Castelli, W.P., Levy, D. (1987). Cholesterol and mortality. 30 years of follow-up from the Framingham study. *JAMA*, **257**: 2176–2180.

Arntzenius, A.C., Kromhout, D., Barth, J.D., *et al.*, (1985). Diet, lipoproteins, and the progression of coronary atherosclerosis. The Leiden Intervention Trial. *N Engl J Med*, **312**: 805–811.

Brady, A.J.B., Betteridge, D.J. (2003). Prevention and risks of treatment with statins. *B J Cardio*, **3**: 218–219.

Cannon CP, Braunwald E, McCabe CH, *et al.*, (2004). Intensive versus moderate lipid lowering with statins after acute coronary syndromes. *N Engl J Med*, **350**: 1495–1504.

Collins, R., Peto, R., Godwin, J., MacMahon, S. (1990) Blood pressure and coronary heart disease. *Lancet*, **336**: 370–371.

De Backer, G., Ambrosioni, E., Borch-Johnsen, K., *et al.*, (2003). European guidelines on cardiovascular disease prevention in clinical practice. Third Joint Task Force of European and Other Societies on Cardiovascular Disease Prevention in Clinical Practice. *Eur Heart J*, **24**: 1601–1610.

Executive Summary of The Third Report of The National Cholesterol Education Program (NCEP) Expert Panel on Detection, Evaluation, And Treatment of High Blood Cholesterol In Adults (Adult Treatment Panel III) (2001). *JAMA*, **285**: 2486–2497.

Greenland, P., Knoll, M.D., Stamler, J., *et al.*, (2003). Major risk factors as antecedents of fatal and nonfatal coronary heart disease. *JAMA*, **290**: 891–897.

Grundy, S.M., Cleeman, J.I., Merz, C.N., *et al.*, (2004). Implications of recent clinical trials for the National Cholesterol Education Program Adult Treatment Panel III guidelines. *Circulation*, **110**: 227–239.

Haffner, S.M., Lehto, S., Ronnemaa, T., *et al.*, (1998). Mortality from coronary heart disease in subjects with type 2 diabetes and in nondiabetic subjects with and without prior myocardial infarction. *N Eng J Med*, **339**: 229–234.

Hansson, L., Zanchetti, A., Carruthers, S.G., *et al.*, (1998). Effects of intensive blood-pressure lowering and low-dose aspirin in patients with hypertension: principal results of the Hypertension Optimal Treatment (HOT) randomized trial. *Lancet* 1998, **351**: 1755–1762.

Heart Protection Study Investigators. (2002). Study of cholesterol lowering with simvastatin in 20,536 high-risk individuals: a randomized placebo-controlled trial. *Lancet*, **360**: 7–22.

JBS 2 (2005): Joint British Societies' guidelines on prevention of cardiovascular disease in clinical practice. *Heart*, **91** Suppl 5: v1–52.

Khot, U.N., Khot, M.B., Bayzer, C.T., et al., (2003). Prevalence of conventional risk factors in patients with coronary heart disease. *JAMA*, **290**: 898–904.

MacMahon, S., Peto, R., Cutler, J., et al., (1990). Blood pressure, stroke, and coronary heart disease. Part 1, Prolonged differences in blood pressure: prospective observational studies corrected for the regression dilution bias. *Lancet*, **335**: 765–774.

Mokdad, A.H., Ford, E.S., Bowman, B.A., et al., (2000). Diabetes trends in the US: 1990–1998. *Diabetes Care*, **23**: 1278–1283.

MRC/BHF Heart Protection Study (2002) of cholesterol lowering with simvastatin in 20,536 high-risk individuals: a randomized placebo-controlled trial. *Lancet*, **360**: 7–22.

MRFIT Study Investigators. (1982). Multiple risk factor intervention trial. Risk factor changes and mortality results. Multiple Risk Factor Intervention Trial Research Group. *JAMA*, **248**: 1465–1477.

Nissen, S.E., Tuzcu, E.M., Schoenhagen, P., et al., (2004). Effect of intensive compared with moderate lipid-lowering therapy on progression of coronary atherosclerosis: a randomized controlled trial. *JAMA*, **291**: 1071–1080.

Ornish, D., Brown, S.E., Scherwitz, L.W., et al., (1990). Can lifestyle changes reverse coronary heart disease? The Lifestyle Heart Trial. *Lancet*, **336**: 129–133.

Primatesta, P., Brookes, M., Poulter, N.R. (2001). Improved hypertension management and control: results from the health survey for England 1998. *Hypertension*, **38**: 827–832.

UK Prospective Diabetes Study (UKPDS) Group (1998). Intensive blood-glucose control with sulphonylureas or insulin compared with conventional treatment and risk of complications in patients with type 2 diabetes (UKPDS 33). *Lancet*, **352**: 837–853.

Verschuren, W.M., Jacobs, D.R., Bloemberg, B.P., et al., (1995). Serum total cholesterol and long-term coronary heart disease mortality in different cultures. Twenty-five-year follow-up of the seven countries study. *JAMA*, **274**:131–136.

Walden, C.E., Retzlaff, B.M., Buck, B.L., et al., (1997). Lipoprotein lipid response to the National Cholesterol Education Program step II diet by hypercholesterolemic and combined hyperlipidemic women and men. *Arterioscler Thromb Vasc Biol*, **17**: 375–382.

Watts, G.F., Lewis, B., Brunt, J.N., et al., (1992). Effects on coronary artery disease of lipid-lowering diet, or diet plus cholestyramine, in the St Thomas' Atherosclerosis Regression Study (STARS). *Lancet*, **339**: 563–569.

Welty, F.K., Stuart, E., O'Meara, M., Huddleston, J. (2002). Effect of addition of exercise to therapeutic lifestyle changes diet in enabling women and men with coronary heart disease to reach Adult Treatment Panel III low-density lipoprotein cholesterol goal without lowering high-density lipoprotein cholesterol. *Am J Cardiol*, **89**: 1201–1304.

West, R., McNeill, A., Raw, M. (2000). Smoking cessation guidelines for health professionals: an update. Health Education Authority. *Thorax*, **55**: 987–999.

Wilson, P.W., D'Agostino, R.B., Levy, D., *et al.*, (1998). Prediction of coronary heart disease using risk factor categories. *Circulation*, **97**: 1837–1847.

Yusuf, S., Hawken, S., Ounpuu, S., *et al.*, (2004). INTERHEART Study Investigators. Effect of potentially modifiable risk factors associated with myocardial infarction in 52 countries (the INTERHEART study): case-control study. *Lancet*, **364**: 937–952.

Chapter 3

Percutaneous Coronary Intervention and Thrombolysis in AMI & other ACS

Frans Visser & Maarten Simoons

Key points

- Acute coronary syndromes (ACS) comprise an evolving acute myocardial infarction (AMI) presenting with or without ST-elevation and unstable angina
- Patients presenting with an ST-elevation MI require immediate reperfusion therapy by primary percutaneous coronary intervention (PCI) or, if such is not available, thrombolysis
- Cardiologists, emergency care physicians, general practitioners and ambulance services should collaborate to develop a national or regional system to optimise AMI therapy, given the national or local facilities and available resources
- A subgroup of high-risk patients presenting with ACS without ST-elevation benefit from PCI or coronary artery bypass graft surgery
- In all patients with ACS intensive anti-platelet and anti-thrombotic therapy is warranted, as well as β-blockers, ACE-inhibitors and statins.

3.1 Introduction

Over the last decades treatment of acute coronary syndromes has dramatically changed from watchful waiting to active interventions to open the occluded infarct artery in case of an ST-elevation myocardial infarction (STEMI) or to intervene early by percutaneous coronary intervention (PCI) or coronary artery bypass graft (CABG) surgery in patients presenting with an acute coronary syndrome without

ST-elevation (non-ST-elevation myocardial infarction – NSTEMI) or unstable angina with high risk features. In this chapter we will focus on thrombolysis and coronary interventions in these two subsets of patients.

3.2 Pathophysiology and clinical presentation

Figure 3.1 depicts the spectrum of clinical presentations in relation to the presence of a non-occluding or occluding thrombus in a coronary artery. Patients with ischaemic chest discomfort may present with or without ST-segment elevation on the ECG. Many patients with such acute coronary syndrome (ACS) will develop myocardial necrosis, and thus a myocardial infarction as recognized by the presence of a serum cardiac marker of necrosis such as CK-MB or a cardiac troponin detected in the blood (Thygesen et al., 2007). Of patients with ST-segment elevation, most will develop a Q-wave infarction (QwMI), while a few develop a non–Q-wave MI (NQMI). Patients who present without ST-segment elevation are suffering from either a non–ST-segment elevation myocardial infarction (NSTEMI) or unstable angina (large open arrows). Most patients presenting with NSTEMI ultimately develop a NQMI on the ECG with a few going on to develop a QwMI. The spectrum ranging from unstable angina through to NSTEMI and STEMI are referred to as the acute coronary syndromes. This chapter will discuss the role of revascularization in patients presenting with STEMI or non-STEMI.

3.3 Early revascularization in STEMI

After sudden coronary occlusion myocardial necrosis develops rapidly. Timely reperfusion therapy salvages myocardium at risk for necrosis, leading to preservation of left ventricular function and ultimately improved survival. The most efficient method for reperfusion is immediate, or direct percutaneous coronary intervention (PCI). Accordingly such treatment is now recommended in European and other guidelines, when available within 1 to 2 hours, provided the intervention can be performed by an experienced team (Van de Werf et al., 2003). The alternative treatment is thrombolysis which can be initiated upon hospital arrival, or preferably pre-hospital by an ambulance crew (paramedics).

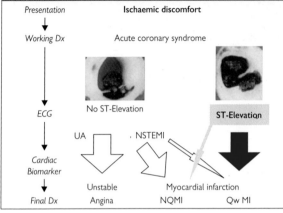

Figure 3.1 Clinical spectrum of presentations of an acute coronary syndrome (Modified from Figure 2 in Antman et al., 2004)

3.4 Primary percutaneous coronary intervention

Primary percutaneous coronary intervention (PPCI) is now considered the treatment of choice in patients presenting with a STEMI. It has been compared with thrombolytic therapy in 23 randomized clinical trials (Keeley et al., 2003). These trials convincingly demonstrate that PPCI treatment results in lower mortality rates, less nonfatal re-infarction and less haemorrhagic stroke compared to thrombolytic therapy (Figure 3.2).

   One important issue with PPCI is the delay between the onset of symptoms and the achievement of myocardial reperfusion. Primary PCI requires transport to hospitals with specialised cardiac intervention facilities and this transport may result in delay of reperfusion therapy. Yet, even in-patients presenting within the first hour after symptom onset, PPCI was demonstrated to be more effective than thrombolysis, in spite of the longer treatment delay for the former therapy (Boersma et al., 2006). Yet, both PPCI as well as thrombolysis are more effective when the delay between the onset of symptoms and reperfusion is shorter (Figure 3.3). Therefore, the European and ACC/AHA guidelines stress the need to lower the recommended medical contact–to-balloon or door-to-balloon time from 120 to 90 minutes in an attempt to maximize the benefits for reperfusion by PPCI (Van de Werf et al., 2003).

Figure 3.2 Clinical outcomes post-STEMI treated with
thrombolytics versus primary percutaneous coronary intervention
(Modified from Figure 2 in Keeley et al., 2003)

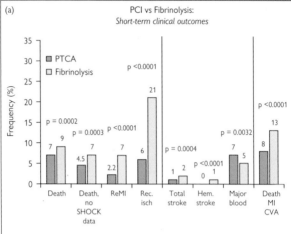

(a) PCI vs Fibrinolysis:
Short-term clinical outcomes

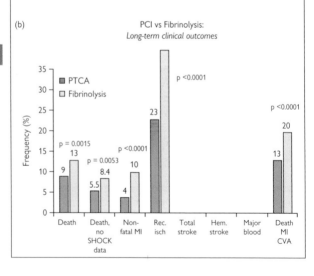

(b) PCI vs Fibrinolysis:
Long-term clinical outcomes

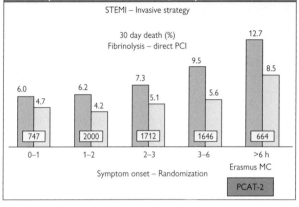

Figure 3.3 Delay between onset of chest symptoms to randomization and 30 day mortality following thrombolysis or PPCI (Data from Boersma et al., 2006)

STEMI – Invasive strategy

30 day death (%)
Fibrinolysis – direct PCI

					12.7
				9.5	8.5
6.0	6.2	7.3		5.6	
4.7	4.2	5.1			
747	2000	1712	1646	664	
0–1	1–2	2–3	3–6	>6 h	

Symptom onset – Randomization

Erasmus MC

PCAT-2

3.4.1 The use of stents in PPCI

Of 22 randomized trials that compared primary PCI with thrombolytic therapy, 12 involved a comparison of primary PCI with stenting and thrombolytic therapy (Boersma *et al.*, 2006). In 9 studies direct stenting was used. The overall results of these investigations were similar as the total group of 22 studies (see above): reduction of mortality, reinfarction and stroke compared to thrombolysis. Compared with balloon angioplasty alone, the use of intracoronary stents resulted in a better immediate angiographic outcome with a larger arterial lumen, less coronary re-occlusion and restenosis of the infarct-related artery, and fewer subsequent myocardial ischaemic events.

The use of drug eluting stents in STEMI patients has been a matter of debate recently. These stents have a similar immediate benefit as bare metal stents, while these reduce in-stent restenosis and the need for re-intervention. However drug eluting stents have also been associated with a slightly increased risk of late stent thrombosis which may cause myocardial infarction and death. The most recent analyses show that drug-eluting stents are associated with similar survival rates after primary PCI compared to bare metal stents (Kastrati *et al.*, 2007). It should be noted that there are important differences among bare metal stents as well as among drug eluting stents. These relate to the stent platform, coating and drug which may be attached. Accordingly it may not be appropriate to lump these together. Large studies are ongoing comparing different stent designs for treatment of stable coronary artery disease as well as ACS.

3.4.2 **PPCI in patients with cardiogenic shock**

In patients with cardiogenic shock, PPCI is recommended. Two relatively small randomized clinical trials (N = 301 and N = 495) have studied the role of PCI in STEMI complicated by cardiogenic shock (Reynolds & Hochman, 2008). Both studies failed to demonstrate a significant reduction in mortality, although in the SHOCK trial there was a significant reduction in mortality in patients less than 75 years of age (Hochman *et al.*, 1999). In the older population with shock, no benefit was apparent, although three registries have demonstrated an improved prognosis in elderly patients who were carefully selected based on clinical data (Reynolds & Hochman, 2008).

3.4.3 **Complications post-PPCI**

Complications of an invasive strategy for treating infarction include:
- complications of the arterial access site (mainly bleeding),
- adverse reactions to volume loading,
- technical complications such as major dissection or perforation of the vessel wall with pericardial haemorrhage,
- excessive bleeding due to anti-platelet and anti-thrombotic therapy,
- renal dysfunction due to the contrast medium,
- coronary reocclusion which occurs in 10% to 15% of patients after PPCI but in less than 5% after stent implantation.

3.4.4 **PPCI in hospitals without surgical back-up**

Due to the increased recognition of PPCI as optimal therapy post-AMI, there are an increasing number of hospitals performing PPCI without surgical back-up. In general, studies on PPCI in these hospitals have shown favourable results. However, PCI in acute infarction does require more experience than routine, elective PCI. Apart from equipment (like the use of an intra-aortic balloon-pump, cooling after prolonged cardiac arrest, ventilator or occasionally haemodialysis), an important component of the success of the intervention is the experience of the operator and the number of interventions that are performed. Therefore, it is recommended that these hospitals do at least a minimum number of primary coronary interventions (ACC/AHA recommendation: at least 36 per year) and that the intervention is performed by an experienced interventional cardiologist (who does at least 75 PCIs per year). In many European countries higher operator volumes (>150 PCI per year) and hospital volumes (>600 procedures per year) are required. Undoubtedly these numbers will change in the coming years.

3.4.5 **Anti-platelet and anti-thrombotic therapy with PPCI**

In addition to aspirin, clopidogrel and heparin, the administration of the GPIIb/IIIa blocker abciximab is recommended with primary PCI because this has been shown to improve clinical outcomes in a recent meta-analysis, although bleeding is more frequent with the combination of these agents (de Luca *et al.*, 2005). A similar benefit was recently shown with bivalirudin, with a lower bleeding rate than with abciximab. The use of fondaparinux with primary PCI is not appropriate since this was associated with increased mortality when compared to heparin (Oldgren *et al.*, 2008). The recently presented TRITON trial demonstrated improved outcomes with the new anti-platelet agent prasugrel compared with heparin (Wiviott *et al.*, 2007). After the procedure, treatment with aspirin should be continued lifelong. Clopidogrel, or when it becomes available prasugrel, should continue for a few months or 1 year or perhaps longer depending on the stent which has been used.

3.5 **Thrombolytic therapy post-AMI**

Thrombolytic therapy is initiated to restore coronary blood flow to the infarcting area by lysis of the occluding clot. There is overwhelming evidence that thrombolysis reduces mortality within 12 hours of onset of infarction (Boersma *et al.*, 1996). Beyond 12 hours there is little evidence for benefit. In patients over 75 years of age the data are conflicting and one registry even showed that in elderly patients the risk of complications surpassed the benefits of thrombolysis. On the other hand a meta-analysis demonstrated a small but significant benefit also in older patients. In general, it is advocated that in older patients thrombolysis is given when mechanical reperfusion is unavailable and when there are no contraindications (Van der Werf *et al.*, 2003). Thrombolytic therapy is combined with other pharmacological agents like anti-platelet therapy (aspirin and clopidogrel), anti-thrombotics (low molecular weight heparin, unfractionated heparin or fondaparinux) as well as statins, β-blockers and ACE inhibitors (Boersma *et al.*, 2003). These are discussed in other chapters of this handbook.

The risks of thrombolytic therapy are related to the lytic activity of the drugs: risk of haemorrhagic stroke (3.9 extra strokes per 1000 treated patients), and major non-cerebral bleeding (4–13% of treated patients) (Boersma *et al.*, 2003; Armstrong *et al.*, 2003). Since patients receive a cocktail of thrombolytic, anti-platelet and anti-coagulant drugs, the bleeding risk can not be attributed to a single agent. In elderly patients, the dose of LMWH should be reduced. Allergic reactions are rare and require appropriate treatment. The contraindications to receiving thrombolytic therapy are listed in Table 3.1.

There are a few thrombolytic agents available: alteplase, reteplase, tenecteplase, and streptokinase. The newer agents alteplase, reteplase and tenecteplase are more effective than streptokinase in achieving

Table 3.1 Contraindications to thrombolytic therapy

Absolute contraindications to thrombolysis

- Haemorrhagic stroke or stroke of unknown origin at any time.
- Ischaemic stroke in the preceding 6 months.
- Central nervous system damage or neoplasms.
- Recent major trauma/surgery/head injury. (within the preceding 3 weeks)
- Gastro-intestinal bleeding within the last month.
- Known bleeding disorder.
- Aortic dissection.

Relative contraindications to thrombolysis

- Transient ischaemic attack in the preceding 6 months.
- Oral anticoagulant therapy.
- Pregnancy or within 1 week post partum.
- Non-compressible punctures.
- Traumatic resuscitation.
- Refractory hypertension (systolic blood pressure >180 mmHg).
- Advanced liver disease.
- Infective endocarditis.
- Active peptic ulcer.

reperfusion but the costs of these drugs are considerably higher and importantly there is an increased risk of intra-cerebral haemorrhage. In the GUSTO trial the net clinical benefit (survival without disabling stroke) was better with alteplase (rtPA) compared with streptokinase (Boersma et al., 2003). Alteplase and tenecteplase have a similar reperfusion efficiency, and a similar incidence of intracerebral hemorrhage, while tenecteplase had significantly lower mild-to-moderate bleeding complications (Van der Werf et al., 2001).

The thrombolytic drugs are combined with aspirin (long-term), clopidogrel (a few days, up to 2 weeks) and low molecular weight heparin (enoxaparin) with an age-adjusted dose. The combination of a thrombolytic with a GPIIb/IIIa blocker has been tested, but appeared to have no benefit over low molecular weight heparin (de Luca et al., 2005). In contrast a recent study with fondaparinux (a specific factor Xa inhibitor) yielded similar efficacy as unfractionated heparin, but with a lower bleeding rate (Oldgren et al., 2008).

3.5.1 Pre-hospital thrombolysis

Randomized controlled trials of thrombolytic therapy have demonstrated the benefit of thrombolytic therapy as early as possible after the onset of infarction (Boersma et al., 1996). It seems reasonable to expect that if thrombolytic therapy could be started at the time of pre-hospital evaluation, a greater number of lives could be saved. Several studies have studied this topic and have showed beneficial trends, although none of the individual trials demonstrated a significant reduction in mortality with pre-hospital initiated thrombolytic therapy. Nevertheless, a meta-analysis of all the available trials clearly demonstrated improved outcome with pre-hospital thrombolytic therapy compared with in-hospital thrombolytic therapy.

Two trials have directly compared pre-hospital thrombolytic therapy with primary percutaneous coronary intervention (PPCI). No clear benefit of pre-hospital thrombolysis was demonstrated, in spite of the longer treatment delay with PPCI (Boersma et al., 2006). Therefore, as PPCI is currently the treatment of choice, the use of pre-hospital thrombolysis can not be advocated for the general population when PPCI is available. However, if the time to admission or to catheterization is significantly delayed, the use of pre-hospital thrombolysis should be considered.

The use of a pre-hospital thrombolytic requires the ability to interpret or to transmit ECG's, paramedic training in ECG interpretation and infarction treatment. Some countries require the presence of a medical supervisor with experience in management of a STEMI, while in other countries the paramedics are sufficiently trained to provide pre-hospital therapy.

3.5.2 **Pre-hospital triage and regional organization**

The choice of reperfusion therapy for patients with MI will depend on regional facilities, in particular the availability of round the clock PCI services, travel distances to hospitals with or without PCI facilities and other resources. It is strongly recommended that a specific protocol is developed in every country/region to optimize care for patients with MI, and particularly to minimize treatment delays. Prehospital recording and interpretation of ECG's facilitates recognition of MI, and significantly reduces treatment delays whether PCI or thrombolysis will be the selected treatment. Hospital based cardiologists, emergency care physicians, general practitioners and ambulance services should work together to optimize MI treatment in their region.

3.6 **PCI for NSTEMI patients**

Coronary revascularization is an integral part of therapeutic approach in high-risk patients with an acute coronary syndrome without ST-elevation (Bassand et al., 2007). Treatment consists of four elements:

1. administration of anti-ischaemic agents,
2. treatment with anticoagulants,
3. administration of antiplatelet therapy and
4. coronary revascularization in selected patients.

The first three are discussed elsewhere in this book. Revascularization is performed to relieve recurrent angina pectoris and ongoing ischaemia and to avoid progression to (extensive) infarction or death. Therefore, angiography and, if appropriate, revascularization should be arranged in patients with persistent angina pectoris or other signs of ischaemia, haemodynamic instability, severe ECG abnormalities or major arrhythmias. In contrast, in patients with low risk of death or infarction, angiography and possible revascularization should be considered only in those patients with stress-induced ischaemia.

The use of systematic early coronary revascularization in all patients presenting with an acute coronary syndrome is still intensely debated. Although several trials showed a favourable trend on mortality or infarction with the direct invasive approach (see Figure 3.4) recent meta-analyses demonstrated a trend towards early excess mortality with the invasive strategy with a long-term survival benefit (Mehta *et al.*, 2005; Qayyum *et al.*, 2008). It should be appreciated that the rates of revascularization achieved in the "early invasive" and "medical or elective invasive" therapy groups varies significantly among the trials. For example, the rate of early intervention in the "invasive" treatment group in the RITA-3 study (44%) was similar to the 40% early revascularization rate in the "elective invasive" group in the recent ICTUS trial (De Winter *et al.*, 2005). On average a strategy of revascularization in about 60% of patients with ACS and without ST-elevation seems to give the best outcome. Therefore the current ESC guidelines recommend a conservative approach in patients who are stabilized on pharmacological therapy and revascularization in selected high risk patients as indicated above (Bassand *et al.*, 2007). In most patients angiography can be deferred until the next working day. Immediate angiography and revascularization is required only in patients with severe ongoing or recurrent ischaemia. After angiography the choice of revascularization, PCI or CABG surgery, is similar to elective procedures and depends on the extent and severity of the lesions, on the condition of the patient and the presence of co-morbidities, and the experience of the interventional and surgical teams.

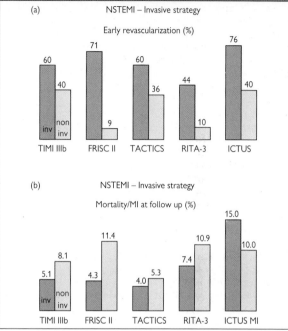

Figure 3.4 Rates of early revascularization and clinical outcomes at one year following an invasive versus conservative strategy

(a) NSTEMI – Invasive strategy

Early revascularization (%)

(b) NSTEMI – Invasive strategy

Mortality/MI at follow up (%)

3.7 Conclusions

In summary, the restoration of coronary perfusion in acute myocardial infarction (STEMI) and the revascularization of critical stenoses in non-ST-elevation acute coronary syndromes, together with intensive pharmacological treatment has profoundly changed the therapeutic approach in patients presenting with an acute coronary syndrome. The invasive strategy has clearly led to improved survival and reduced complication rates. A summary of the various treatment strategies used in the management of ACS is presented in Figure 3.5.

Figure 3.5 A summary of the treatment strategies used in ACS

ACS	No-ST↑		ST↑		
Combine	Med	PCI	PCI	lysis	none
Aspirin					
Clopidogrel					
IIb/IIIa bl.					
Select					
UF Heparin					
LMWH					
Fondapar					
Bivalirudin					

your choice

Key references

Antman, E.M., Anbe, D.T., Armstrong, P.W., et al., (2004). ACC/AHA guidelines for the management of patients with ST-elevation myocardial infarction; A report of the American College of Cardiology/American Heart Association Task Force on Practice Guidelines (Committee to Revise the 1999 Guidelines for the Management of patients with acute myocardial infarction). J Am Coll Cardiol, 44: E1–E211.

Armstrong, P.W., Collen, D., Antman, E.M., et al., (2003). Fibrinolysis for acute myocardial infarction. The future is here and now. Circulation, 107: 2533–2537.

Bassand, J.P., Hamm, C.W., Ardissino, D., et al., (2007). The Task Force for the diagnosis and treatment of non-ST-segment elevation acute coronary syndromes of the European Society of Cardiology. Guidelines for the diagnosis and treatment of non-ST-segment elevation acute coronary syndromes. Eur Heart J, 28: 15989–1660.

Boersma, E., Maas, A.C., Deckers, J.W., et al., (1996). Early thrombolytic treatment in acute myocardial infarction: reappraisal of the golden hour. Lancet, 348: 771–775.

Boersma, E., Mercado, N., Poldermans, D., et al., (2003). Acute myocardial infarction. Lancet, 361: 847–858.

Boersma, E. (2006). The Primary Coronary Angioplasty vs. Thrombolysis Group. Does time matter? A pooled analysis of randomized clinical trials comparing primary percutaneous coronary intervention and in-hospital fibrinolysis in acute myocardial infarction patients. Eur Heart J, 27: 779–788.

De Luca, G, Suryapranata, H., Stone, G.W., *et al.*, (2005). Abciximab as adjunctive therapy to reperfusion in acute ST-segment elevation myocardial infarction. A meta-analysis of randomized trials. *JAMA*, **293**: 1759–1765.

De Winter, R.J., Windhausen, F., Cornel, J.H., *et al.*, (2005). Early invasive versus selectively invasive management for acute coronary syndromes. *N Engl J Med*, **353**: 1095–1104.

Hochman, J.S., Sleeper, L.A., Webb, J.G., *et al.*, (1999). Early revascularization in acute myocardial infarction compli-cated by cardiogenic shock: SHOCK Investigators: Should we emergently revascularize occluded coronaries for cardiogenic shock. *N Engl J Med*, **341**: 625–634.

Kastrati, A., Dibra, A., Spaulding, C., *et al.*, (2007). Meta-analysis of randomized trials on drug-eluting stents vs bare-metal stents in patients with acute myocardial infarction. *Eur Heart J*, **28**: 2706–2713.

Keeley, E.C., Boura, J.A., Grines, C.L. (2003). Primary angioplasty versus intravenous thrombolytic therapy for acute myocardial infarction: a quantitative review of 23 randomized trials. *Lancet*, **361**: 13–20.

Mehta, S.R., Cannon, C.P., Fox, K.A.A., *et al.*, (2005). Routine vs selective invasive strategies in patients with acute coronary syndromes. A collaborative meta-analysis of randomized trials. *JAMA*, **293**: 2908–2917.

Oldgren, J., Wallentin, L., Afzal, R., *et al.*, (2008) Effects of fondaparinux on mortality and reinfarction in patients with acute ST-segment elevation myocardial infarction. The OASIS-6 randomized trial. *JAMA*, **295**: 1519–1530.

Qayyum, R., Khalid, M.R., Andomaityte, J. (2008). Systematic review: comparing routine and selective invasive strategies for the acute coronary syndrome. *Ann Intern Med*, **148**: 186–196.

Reynolds, H.R., Hochman, J.S. (2008). Cardiogenic shock. Current concepts and improving outcomes. *Circulation*, **117**: 686–697.

Thygesen, K., Alpert, J.S., White, H.D. (2007). Universal definition of myocardial infarction. On behalf of the Joint ESC/ACCF/AHA/WHF Task Force for the redefinition of myocardial infarction. *Eur Heart J*, **28**: 2525–2538.

Van de Werf, F., Barron, H.V., Armstrong P.L., *et al.*, (2001). Incidence and predictors of bleeding events after fibrinolytic therapy with fibrin-specific agents. A comparison of TNK-tPA and rt-PA. *Eur Heart J*, **22**: 2253–2261.

Van de Werf, F., Ardissino, D., Betriu, A., *et al.*, (2003). Management of acute myocardial infarction in patients presenting with ST-segment elevation. The Task force on the management of acute myocardial infarction of the European society of Cardiology. *Eur Heart J*, **24**: 28–66.

Wiviott, S.D., Braunwald, E, McCabe, C.H., *et al.*, (2007). Prasugrel versus Clopidogrel in patients with acute coronary syndromes. *N Engl J Med*, **357**: 2001–2015.

Chapter 4

Anti-Platelet and Anti-Thrombotic Therapy Post-AMI

Dana Dawson & Keith Fox

Key points

- Acute coronary syndromes (ACS) encompass a spectrum of presentations which include unstable angina, non-ST-elevation myocardial infarction (NSTEMI or NSTE-ACS), and ST-elevation myocardial infarction (STEMI or STE-ACS)
- Anti-platelet and anti-thrombotic agents are administered as ancillary therapy to myocardial reperfusion in patients presenting with an acute coronary syndrome, to maintain the patency of the infarct-related coronary artery
- More specific and potent inhibitors of platelet activation and of the coagulation cascade are emerging with the aim being to further improve clinical outcomes in patients presenting with an acute coronary syndrome, without increasing the risks of major bleeding.

4.1 Background

Coronary heart disease (CHD) is the single leading cause of morbidity and mortality and an important economic burden. All acute coronary syndromes (ACS) share a common pathology: the disruption of the cholesterol-rich atherosclerotic plaque which erodes, fissures or ruptures, leading to platelet aggregation, thrombus formation and distal embolisation. This results in varying degrees of myocardial ischaemia which manifest in ACS as chest pain. The clinical diagnosis is confirmed by the ECG (which can be normal or show ST deviation or T wave changes) and the measurement of troponins, as highlighted in the recent ESC guidelines (Bassand et al., 2007). Non ST-elevation ACS (NSTE-ACS) has become the predominant presentation compared with ST-elevation ACS for various reasons that include better diagnostic tools and biomarker sensitivity.

In the absence of a therapeutic cardioprotective regimen at the time of presentation with ACS, the aim of current treatment strategies is to spare cardiomyocytes that remain viable in the coronary territory subtended by the culprit lesion. In contrast, endogenous cardioprotective mechanisms may have been initiated in the prodrome of the syndrome, in the context of repetitive ischaemic episodes, and may be amplified by therapeutic agents administered for other indications (myocardial 'preconditioning', see Chapter 8). Effective cardioprotective agents are important in NSTE-ACS as the mortality of such patients eventually matches or exceeds that of patients presenting with ST-elevation MI (within 6–12 months) (Terkelsen et al., 2005). The immediate treatment of ACS aims to reduce myocardial ischaemia, inhibit platelet aggregation and further thrombus formation and to improve tissue perfusion with mechanical revascularization (usually percutaneous coronary intervention, PCI). Depending on the extent and complications of ischaemia, patients undergo emergency or early elective (within about 72 hours) coronary angiography and PCI to reduce obstruction at the site of the disrupted and thrombosed coronary artery.

A meta-analysis of randomized trials has shown that a routine invasive approach is associated with less early cardiovascular morbidity and mortality (death or MI) and reduced refractory ischaemia compared with those in whom a selective invasive approach was taken (Mehta et al., 2005). Furthermore, long term follow-up data demonstrates a sustained benefit of an early invasive strategy in patients with NSTE-ACS at moderate to high risk (Lagerqvist et al., 2006). Anti-thrombotic regimens are effective in reducing thrombus growth on the disrupted plaque and platelet aggregation and in reducing acute complications including ischaemia and myocardial infarction. However, in the absence of revascularization no medical regimen has been successful, so far, in reducing major complications (death and MI) in the medium or longer term, nor in stimulating regression of the atherosclerotic burden.

4.2 Anti-Platelet therapy

Activated platelets are critical in the pathophysiological mechanisms following acute plaque disruption and in the perpetuation of thrombus formation. Indirect 'Cardioprotection', which manifests as improved clinical outcomes of patients with ACS, has been achieved by the inhibition of platelet activation and aggregation. Current anti-platelet therapies include:

1. irreversible cyclo-oxygenase-1 inhibitors which inhibit the release of Thromboxane A2 by the thrombocyte, thus decreasing platelet activation (e.g. aspirin);

2. thienopyridines, which inhibit ADP receptor-mediated platelet activation and aggregation (e.g. clopidogrel, prasugrel and ticlopidine);

3. glycoprotein (GP) IIb/IIIa inhibitors, which inhibit fibrinogen and vWF binding to the IIb/IIIa receptor of activated adherent platelets to prevent platelet aggregation (e.g. abciximab, tirofiban and eptifibatide); and

4. inhibitors of the thrombin platelet receptor.

4.2.1 **Aspirin**

The most extensively tested drug, for which the most compelling evidence to date exists, is aspirin. The ISIS-2 (The Second International Study of Infarct Survival) (Baigent *et al.*, 1998) trial has shown clear benefit at ten years of those treated with aspirin after a STE-ACS and further data supports its protective role in NSTE-ACS. Aspirin is given as a loading dose of 300 mg followed by daily maintenance of 75 mg, life-long. Aspirin resistance is rare, contraindications are allergy and bleeding disorders, in which case aspirin can be empirically substituted with clopidogrel.

4.2.2 **Thienopyridines**

The beneficial effects of adding clopidogrel to aspirin were reported in the CURE trial (Yusuf *et al.*, 2001), in which patients with ACS were randomized to receive a loading dose of 300 mg of clopidogrel followed by 75 mg daily maintenance dose. The arm assigned to clopidogrel therapy had a decreased risk of subsequent coronary ischaemia and cardiovascular death, MI or stroke compared to placebo (RR 0.8, 95% CI 0.72 to 0.9, p<0.01). The benefit of dual anti-platelet therapy was confirmed for up to 1 and 3 years in the CREDO (Early and sustained dual oral antiplatelet therapy following percutaneous coronary intervention: a randomized controlled trial) and CAPRIE (A randomized, blinded, trial of clopidogrel versus aspirin in patients at risk of ischaemic events) trials (Steinbuhl *et al.*, 2002; CAPRIE Study Investigators 1996). This benefit is sustained in those undergoing PCI in the setting of NSTE-ACS (Mehta *et al.*, 2001; Steinbuhl *et al.*, 2002). Loading dose with 300 mg clopidogrel achieves effective platelet inhibition in 4–6 hours, whereas a higher loading dose of 600 mg achieves the same level of platelet inhibition after 2 hours, although non-responders to clopidogrel have been identified. Treatment with clopidogrel in addition to aspirin raises the risk of bleeding (approx 1% excess major bleeds) and this risk has recently shown to be higher with the newer generation thienopyridine, prasugrel, in the context of more potent platelet inhibition (Wiviott *et al.*, 2007).

Recent clinical studies have reported benefit with clopidogrel added to aspirin in patients presenting with a STE-ACS. In the COMMIT-CCS-2

STUDY, Chen et al., (2005) reported that the addition of clopidogrel 75 mg daily reduced by 9%, the primary combined end-point of death, reinfarction or stroke in (2121 [9.2%] clopidogrel vs 2310 [10.1%] placebo; p = 0.002), in 21.353 patients presenting with a STEMI or bundle branch block. The CLARITY-TIMI 28 trial reported that the addition of clopidogrel (300 mg oral loading dose plus 75 mg daily maintenance dose) reduced the primary composite endpoint of an occluded infarct artery, death or recurrent MI by 6.7% in STEMI patients (18–75 years) receiving reperfusion with thrombolytic therapy (Sabatine et al., 2005).

The updated ACC/AHA guidelines for the management of patients with STEMI (Antman et al., 2008) recommends an oral loading dose of 300 mg clopidogrel followed by 75 mg daily maintenance therapy for 1 year in patients (<75 years) presenting with a STEMI regardless of whether they received reperfusion using thrombolytics or not (Class IIA recommendation).

4.2.3 Glycoprotein IIb/IIIa inhibitors

Abciximab is a monoclonal antibody directed at the glycoprotein (GP) IIb-IIIa receptor; tirofiban and eptifibatide are synthetic molecules that mimic an amino-acid sequence to which fibrinogen binds in the formation of thrombus. In patients with NSTE-ACS, several trials have reported benefit with the addition of tirofiban (Platelet Receptor Inhibition for Ischaemic Syndrome Management in Patients Limited by Unstable Signs and Symptoms – PRISM-PLUS and Platelet Receptor Inhibition in Ischemic Syndrome Management – PRISM) (Zhao et al., 1999; PRISM Study Investigators 1998) or eptifibatide (PURSUIT Study Investigators 1998) to aspirin and heparin in terms of a reduction in the composite end point of early death, nonfatal myocardial infarction and refractory ischaemia. Following these first two trials which have demonstrated the beneficial effects of adding a GP IIb-IIIa inhibitor to unfractionated heparin, the PARAGON-B study (Platelet IIb/IIIa Antagonist for the Reduction of Acute coronary syndrome events in a Global Organization Network B) found that the combination of aspirin, GP IIB/IIIa inhibitors and low molecular weight heparins (LMWH) was safe and had the same reduction effect in refractory ischaemia. Evidence of higher mortality emerged from GUSTO-IV-ACS trial, which randomized patients (without PCI) to abciximab versus placebo in addition to aspirin and/without heparin. This adverse effect (also seen with oral IIb/IIa inhibitors) was thought to have occurred due to low levels of platelet inhibition which may have a paradoxical pro-thrombotic effect (via CD40 ligand shedding from platelets at sub-threshold GP IIb/IIIa blockade), at the dose administered in this study. Combined data from all randomized studies using GP IIb/IIIa inhibitors in NSTE-ACS patients without PCI (PRISM, PRISM-PLUS, PARAGON, PARAGON-A, PARAGON-B, PURSUIT and GUSTO-IV) are disappointing, as there is only a modest

8.5% relative reduction in 30-day composite end-point of death/MI. This small benefit is in contrast with the overall early relative reduction of 38% in death/MI offered by the use of GP IIb/IIIa inhibitors in the setting of elective PCI. In addition, trials are on going with regard to the exact timing of GP IIb/IIIa therapy. Recently, studies using bivalirudin (a direct thrombin inhibitor – see below) have shown similar efficacy and reduced bleeding compared with and IIb/IIIa inhibitor plus aspirin. In summary, the GP IIb/IIIa inhibitors have failed to provide protection outside the setting of PCI in NSTE-ACS and STE-ACS treated with primary PCI (Stone *et al.*, 2002; Montalescot *et al.*, 2001).

4.3 Anti-thrombotic therapy

A second and potent cardio-protective mechanism in NSTE-ACS is through the inhibition of the coagulation cascade or by directly inhibiting thrombin. There are several targets for such pharmacotherapy in the intrinsic and common coagulation pathways. These are:

1. unfractionated heparin (UFH), an indirect inhibitor via anti-thrombin III;
2. low molecular weight heparins (LMWH: enoxaparin, dalteparin) which inhibit Factor IIa (activated thrombin) and mainly Factor Xa to preventing both the action and generation of further thrombin;
3. direct thrombin inhibitors (hirudin, the DNA recombinant analogue lepirudin and the synthetic analogue bivalirudin) which bind directly to thrombin;
4. indirect (fondaparinux) or direct oral Xa inhibitors; and
5. platelet thrombin receptor antagonists are in development and clinical testing.

41

4.3.1 Unfractionated heparin

Unfractionated heparin (UFH) provided the first anticoagulation treatment in NSTE-ACS and has a rapid onset of action when administered parenterally. However it is difficult to maintain anticoagulation within the therapeutic range, and the cessation of UFH can be followed by rebound activation. Aspirin plus UFH results in lower death/MI rates compared to aspirin alone in patients with unstable angina (Theroux *et al.*, 1993). The dose administered is 5000 units as an intravenous bolus followed by a continuous infusion aiming to maintain an activated partial thromboplastin time (APTT) between 1.5–2.5 times control. This requires frequent monitoring of the APTT and infusion dose adjustment.

4.3.2 **Low molecular weight heparins**

Low molecular weight heparins (LMWHs) have several advantages over UFH: they are less likely to induce thrombocytopenia and are more potent inhibitors of Factor Xa, thereby providing better thrombin inhibition. As these depolymerized, small molecules are circulating free, rather than bound to plasma proteins, they provide more consistent anticoagulation and obviate the need for monitoring. They are eliminated through the kidneys and patients with marked renal dysfunction run the risk of over anticoagulation, hence in such patients the administration of UFH with frequent monitoring is still advocated. Several trials have demonstrated the superiority of LMWH compared to aspirin alone or compared to aspirin plus UFH. The Fragmin during Instability in Coronary Artery Disease (FRISC) study group demonstrated the superiority of subcutaneous dalteparin versus placebo in patients with NSTE-ACS otherwise receiving aspirin and standard anti-anginal treatment. The Fragmin in unstable coronary artery disease (FRIC) study provided evidence that LMWH may be an alternative to UFH in the acute treatment of NSTE-ACS, by comparing twice daily subcutaneous dalteparin *versus* UFH in combination with aspirin. In the first 6 days, the rate of death, myocardial infarction, or recurrence of angina was reduced, but the effect was not sustained after discontinuation. A meta-analysis of randomized trials comparing UFH or LMWH with placebo or untreated control, or comparing UFH with LMWH, for the short-term and long-term management comprising 17157 patients with NSTE-ACS concluded that there was similar efficacy and safety of LMWH and UFH (Eikelboom et al., 2000). An exception to this conclusion appears to be the use of enoxaparin and the ESSENCE (Efficacy and Safety of Subcutaneous Enoxaparin in Non-Q-Wave Coronary Events Study Group) (Cohen et al., 1997), TIMI 11B (Enoxaparin prevents death and cardiac ischemic events in unstable angina/non-Q-wave myocardial infarction) clinical trials. Results of the thrombolysis in myocardial infarction (TIMI) 11B trial clearly demonstrated that the administration of enoxaparin in addition to aspirin was more effective than UFH plus aspirin in reducing the incidence of ischaemic events in patients with NSTE-ACS. High risk patients (those with ST-segment changes on the 12-lead ECG and those with elevated Troponin I levels) appear to derive the highest benefit in both studies. Furthermore, a marked benefit of enoxaparin treatment was noted in those undergoing PCI (Fox et al., 2002; White et al., 2006). To summarize, the use of enoxaparin in addition to GP IIb/IIIa inhibitors and aspirin is safe. In the CREATE trial, Yusuf et al., (2005) reported that reviparin reduced mortality and reinfarction in patients presenting with STE-ACS, without a significant increase in overall stroke rates, although there was a small absolute excess of life-threatening bleeding.

4.3.3 **Direct thrombin inhibitors**

Hirudin, the prototypical direct thrombin inhibitor, is a naturally occurring polypeptide found in leech saliva. The Global Use of Strategies to Open Occluded Coronary Arteries (Gusto-IIb) trial compared hirudin and heparin in patients with NSTE-ACS or acute STE-MI, but did not show improved efficacy with the direct thrombin inhibitor (Metz et al., 1998). The OASIS-2 study (Effects of recombinant hirudin [lepirudin] versus heparin in patients without ST-elevation) showed early benefit, but this was not sustained and there was excess bleeding (OASIS-2 Trial Investigators 1999). The ACUITY trial (Antithrombotic strategies in patients with acute coronary syndromes undergoing early invasive management) assigned patients to heparin plus GP IIb/IIIa inhibitors, bivalirudin plus GP IIb/IIIa inhibitors, or bivalirudin monotherapy (Stone et al., 2006). The early results of this randomized study showed no statistically significant difference in rates of composite ischaemia or mortality among patients with moderate- and high-risk NSTE-ACS undergoing invasive treatment with the 3 different therapies. Anticoagulation with bivalirudin alone suppresses adverse ischaemic events to a similar extent as does heparin plus glycoprotein IIb/IIIa inhibitors, while significantly lowering the risk of major haemorrhagic complications. Thus direct thrombin inhibitors, in particular bivalirudin, have the potential to emerge as equivalent therapy to enoxaparin or UFH plus GP IIb/IIIa for patients with NSTE-ACS.

4.3.4 **Oral Xa inhibitors**

The OASIS-5 trial (Efficacy and safety of fondaparinux versus enoxaparin in patients with acute coronary syndromes undergoing PCI) compared fondaparinux with enoxaparin (Mehta et al., 2007). Fondaparinux, which is a synthetic pentasaccharide that inhibits factor Xa by binding to antithrombin, reduced major bleeding by more than one-half (2.4% vs. 5.1%, hazard ratio [HR] 0.46, p <0.00001) at day 9, with similar rates of ischaemic events, resulting in superior net clinical benefit (death, myocardial infarction, stroke, major bleeding: 8.2% vs. 10.4%, HR 0.78, p = 0.004). A concern was that catheter thrombus was more common in patients receiving fondaparinux (0.9%) than enoxaparin alone (0.4%), but this was largely prevented by using UFH at the time of PCI, without any increase in bleeding. The benefits of fondaparinux over enoxaparin when administered for NSTE-ACS are most marked among patients with renal dysfunction and are largely explained by lower rates of major bleeding with fondaparinux (Fox et al., 2007). In the OASIS-6 study (Yusuf et al., 2006), fondaparinux was found to reduce mortality and reinfarction without increasing bleeding and strokes in STE-ACS patients, particularly those not undergoing primary percutaneous coronary intervention.

4.4 Conclusions

The combination of anti-platelet agents, anti-coagulants and invasive coronary procedures aims to protect the myocardium against ischaemic events in patients presenting with an acute coronary syndrome, by maintaining the patency of the infarct-related coronary artery. More specific and potent inhibition of platelet activation and of the coagulation cascade aims to improve efficacy without increasing the risks of major bleeding. However, none of these agents specifically protect the myocardium from injury, rather they improve myocardial perfusion and reduce the ischaemic burden. Therefore, these agents need to be used in conjunction with adjunctive therapy which specifically protects cardiomyocytes against ischaemia-reperfusion injury (see Chapters 8 and 9).

Key references

Antman, E.M., Hand, M., Armstrong, P.W., et al., (2008). 2007 focused update of the ACC/AHA 2004 guidelines for the management of patients with ST-elevation myocardial infarction: a report of the American College of Cardiology/American Heart Association Task Force on Practice Guidelines. *J Am Coll Cardiol*, **51**: 210–247.

Baigent, C., Collins, R., Appleby, P., et al., (1998). ISIS-2: 10 year survival among patients with suspected acute myocardial infarction in randomized comparison of intravenous streptokinase, oral aspirin, both, or neither. The ISIS-2 (Second International Study of Infarct Survival) Collaborative Group. *BMJ*, **316**: 1337–1343.

Bassand, J.P., Hamm, C.W., Ardissino, D., et al., (2007). Guidelines for the diagnosis and treatment of non-ST-segment elevation acute coronary syndromes. *Eur Heart J*, **28**: 1598–1660.

CAPRIE Study Investigators. (1996). A randomized, blinded, trial of clopidogrel versus aspirin in patients at risk of ischaemic events (CAPRIE). CAPRIE Steering Committee. *Lancet*, **348**: 1329–1339.

Chen, Z.M., Jiang, L.X., Chen, Y.P., et al., (2005). Addition of clopidogrel to aspirin in 45,852 patients with acute myocardial infarction: randomized placebo-controlled trial. *Lancet*, **366**: 1607–1621.

Cohen, M., Demers, C., Gurfinkel, E.P., et al., (1997). A comparison of low-molecular-weight heparin with unfractionated heparin for unstable coronary artery disease. Efficacy and Safety of Subcutaneous Enoxaparin in Non-Q-Wave Coronary Events Study Group. *N Engl J Med*, **337**: 447–452.

Eikelboom, J.W., Anand, S.S., Malmberg, K., et al., (2000). Unfractionated heparin and low-molecular-weight heparin in acute coronary syndrome without ST-elevation: a meta-analysis. *Lancet*, **355**: 1936–1942.

Fox, K.A., Antman, E.M., Cohen, M., Bigonzi, F. (2002). Comparison of enoxaparin versus unfractionated heparin in patients with unstable angina pectoris/non-ST-segment elevation acute myocardial infarction having subsequent percutaneous coronary intervention. *Am J Cardiol*, **90**: 477–482.

Fox, K.A., Bassand, J.P., Mehta, S.R, *et al.*, (2007). Influence of renal function on the efficacy and safety of fondaparinux relative to enoxaparin in non ST-segment elevation acute coronary syndromes. *Ann Intern Med*, **147**: 304–310.

Lagerqvist, B., Husted, S., Kontny, F., *et al.*, (2006). 5-year outcomes in the FRISC-II randomized trial of an invasive versus a non-invasive strategy in non-ST-elevation acute coronary syndrome: a follow-up study. *Lancet*, **368**: 998–1004.

Mehta, S.R., Yusuf, S., Peters, R.J., *et al.*, (2001). Effects of pretreatment with clopidogrel and aspirin followed by long-term therapy in patients undergoing percutaneous coronary intervention: the PCI-CURE study. *Lancet*, **358**: 527–533.

Mehta, S.R., Cannon, C.P., Fox, K.A., *et al.*, (2005). Routine vs selective invasive strategies in patients with acute coronary syndromes: a collaborative meta-analysis of randomized trials. *JAMA*, **293**: 2908–2917.

Mehta, S.R., Granger, C.B., Eikelboom, J.W., *et al.*, (2007). Efficacy and safety of fondaparinux versus enoxaparin in patients with acute coronary syndromes undergoing percutaneous coronary intervention: results from the OASIS-5 trial. *J Am Coll Cardiol* 2007, **50**: 1742–1751.

Metz, B.K., White, H.D., Granger, C.B., *et al.*, (1998). Randomized comparison of direct thrombin inhibition versus heparin in conjunction with fibrinolytic therapy for acute myocardial infarction: results from the GUSTO-IIb Trial. Global Use of Strategies to Open Occluded Coronary Arteries in Acute Coronary Syndromes (GUSTO-IIb) Investigators. *J Am Coll Cardiol*, **31**: 1493–1498.

Montalescot, G., Barragan, P., Wittenberg, O., *et al.*, (2001). Platelet glycoprotein IIb/IIIa inhibition with coronary stenting for acute myocardial infarction. *N Engl J Med*, **344**: 1895–1903.

PARAGON Study Investigators. (1998). International, randomized, controlled trial of lamifiban (a platelet glycoprotein IIb/IIIa inhibitor), heparin, or both in unstable angina. The PARAGON Investigators. Platelet IIb/IIIa Antagonism for the Reduction of Acute coronary syndrome events in a Global Organization Network. *Circulation*, **97**: 2386–2395.

PRISM Study Investigators. (1998). A comparison of aspirin plus tirofiban with aspirin plus heparin for unstable angina. Platelet Receptor Inhibition in Ischemic Syndrome Management (PRISM) Study Investigators. *N Engl J Med*, **338**: 1498–1505.

PURSUIT Study Investigators. (1998). Inhibition of platelet glycoprotein IIb/IIIa with eptifibatide in patients with acute coronary syndromes. The PURSUIT Trial Investigators. Platelet Glycoprotein IIb/IIIa in Unstable Angina: Receptor Suppression Using Integrilin Therapy. *N Engl J Med*, **339**: 436–443.

Sabatine, M.S., Cannon, C.P., Gibson, C.M., et al., (2005). Addition of clopidogrel to aspirin and fibrinolytic therapy for myocardial infarction with ST-segment elevation. N Engl J Med, **352**: 1179–1189.

Steinhubl, S.R., Berger, P.B., Mann, J.T. III, et al., (2002). Early and sustained dual oral antiplatelet therapy following percutaneous coronary intervention: a randomized controlled trial. JAMA, **288**: 2411–2420.

Stone, G.W., Grines, C.L., Cox, D.A., et al., (2002). Comparison of angioplasty with stenting, with or without abciximab, in acute myocardial infarction. N Engl J Med, **346**: 957–966.

Stone, G.W., McLaurin, B.T., Cox, D.A., et al., (2006). Bivalirudin for patients with acute coronary syndromes. N Engl J Med, **355**: 2203–2216.

Terkelsen, C.J., Lassen, J.F., Norgaard, B.L., et al., (2005). Mortality rates in patients with ST-elevation vs. non-ST-elevation acute myocardial infarction: observations from an unselected cohort. Eur Heart J, **26**: 18–26.

Theroux, P., Waters, D., Qiu, S., et al., (1993). Aspirin versus heparin to prevent myocardial infarction during the acute phase of unstable angina. Circulation, **88**: 2045–2048.

White, H.D., Kleiman, N.S., Mahaffey, K.W., et al., (2006). Efficacy and safety of enoxaparin compared with unfractionated heparin in high-risk patients with non-ST-segment elevation acute coronary syndrome undergoing percutaneous coronary intervention in the Superior Yield of the New Strategy of Enoxaparin, Revascularization and Glycoprotein IIb/IIIa Inhibitors (SYNERGY) trial. Am Heart J, **152**: 1042–1050.

Wiviott, S.D., Braunwald, E., McCabe, C.H., et al., (2007). Prasugrel versus clopidogrel in patients with acute coronary syndromes. N Engl J Med, **357**: 2001–2015.

Yusuf, S., Zhao, F., Mehta, S.R., et al., (2001). Effects of clopidogrel in addition to aspirin in patients with acute coronary syndromes without ST-segment elevation. N Engl J Med, **345**: 494–502.

Yusuf, S., Mehta, S.R., Xie, C., et al., (2005). Effects of reviparin, a low-molecular-weight heparin, on mortality, reinfarction, and strokes in patients with acute myocardial infarction presenting with ST-segment elevation. JAMA, **293**: 427–435.

Yusuf, S., Mehta, S.R., Chrolavicius, S., et al., (2006). Effects of fondaparinux on mortality and reinfarction in patients with acute ST-segment elevation myocardial infarction: the OASIS-6 randomized trial. JAMA, **295**: 1519–1530.

Zhao, X.Q., Theroux, P., Snapinn, SM., Sax, F.L. (1999). Intracoronary thrombus and platelet glycoprotein IIb/IIIa receptor blockade with tirofiban in unstable angina or non-Q-wave myocardial infarction. Angiographic results from the PRISM-PLUS trial (Platelet receptor inhibition for ischemic syndrome management in patients limited by unstable signs and symptoms). PRISM-PLUS Investigators. Circulation, **100**: 1609–1615.

Chapter 5

Coronary No-Reflow and Microvascular Obstruction

Derek Hausenloy & Derek Yellon

Key points

- Following an AMI, the restoration of TIMI III coronary blood flow using thrombolytic therapy or primary percutaneous coronary intervention does not guarantee actual myocardial perfusion
- In 40–60% of reperfused AMI cases, myocardial perfusion is impeded at the level of the capillaries due to microvascular obstruction (MVO)- a phenomenon termed coronary no-reflow
- The presence of coronary no-reflow can be detected as impaired myocardial perfusion using non-invasive imaging modalities such as nuclear myocardial perfusion scanning, myocardial contrast echocardiography or contrast-enhanced cardiac magnetic resonance imaging
- The presence of microvascular obstruction post-AMI is associated with a larger infarct size, impaired LV ejection fraction, adverse LV remodelling and poorer clinical outcomes
- Current treatment strategies include; vasodilator therapy such as adenosine, calcium-channel blockers, and nitrates; distal protection to prevent microemboli; and glycoprotein IIb/IIIa inhibitors
- Novel treatment strategies are required to prevent and treat coronary no-reflow, thereby improving myocardial perfusion, reducing myocardial infarct size, preserving LV ejection fraction, preventing LV remodeling and improving clinical outcomes.

5.1 Definition of no-reflow and MVO

It is well-established that following a ST-elevation myocardial infarction (STEMI), rapidly establishing and maintaining a patent coronary artery is the most effective means of salvaging viable myocardium and limiting infarct size. However, although TIMI III unobstructed coronary flow may be achieved on angiography, this does not guarantee actual perfusion of the previously ischaemic myocardium, given the existence of coronary 'no-reflow', a process which results from microvascular obstruction, a complex phenomenon characterized by impedance to microvascular blood flow, encountered on opening the infarct-related coronary artery (Ito, 2006; van Gaal & Banning, 2007).

The 'no-reflow' phenomenon was first described as the 'inability to reperfuse a previously ischemic region' by Krug and colleagues in 1966 using a feline model of myocardial ischaemia-reperfusion injury (Krug et al., 1966). Its ultrastructural features were later characterized in the reperfused canine heart by Kloner and colleagues in 1974 (Kloner et al., 1974). Despite intensive research, the actual cause of the no-reflow phenomenon remains unclear although the major contributory factors are thought to include capillary damage with impaired vasodilatation, external capillary compression by endothelial cell and cardiomyocyte swelling, microembolization of friable material released from the atherosclerotic plaque, platelet microthrombi, and neutrophil plugging (Kloner et al., 1974; Ito 2006; van Gaal & Banning, 2007).

Microvascular obstruction is a phenomenon which manifests at the onset of myocardial reperfusion and which follows a sustained episode of acute myocardial ischaemia. It is an acute phenomenon which develops over the first 48 hrs following reperfusion and lasts up to about 3 months (Rochitte et al., 1998). In reperfused STEMI patients, it has been reported that the development of the MVO is determined by several factors which include, amongst others, the extent of myocardial injury, and the size of the myocardium at risk of infarction (Iwakura et al., 2001).

5.2 Clinical significance of MVO

Coronary no-reflow may affect between 30–60% of reperfused STEMI patients depending on the imaging modality used to detect its presence with cardiac MRI being the most sensitive technique. Patients experiencing particularly severe no-reflow experience chest pain, persistent ST-elevation and hemodynamic compromise in the cardiac catheter laboratory. Its presence as detected by myocardial contrast echocardiography, contrast enhanced cardiac MRI or angiographic markers of no-reflow is associated with a larger myocardial infarct size, worse LV ejection fraction, adverse LV remodelling and worse short-term and long-term clinical outcomes (Wu et al., 1998; De Luca et al., 2004). The ability to detect and quantify this phenomenon in reperfused STEMI patients is now possible with recent advances in non-invasive imaging techniques, which makes feasible the identification of high-risk patients who may benefit from more intensive treatment to either prevent or treat coronary no-reflow.

5.3 Detecting MVO post-AMI

There are several methods available for detecting coronary reflow either in the catheter laboratory at the time of primary percutaneous coronary intervention (PPCI) or its presence may be indicated by a myocardial perfusion defect on subsequent non-invasive imaging, reflecting underlying MVO.

5.3.1 Detecting MVO at the time of PPCI

There are several methods available at the time of PCI which can be used to indicate the presence of no-reflow in reperfused STEMI patients. The success of PPCI is usually indicated by the presence of a patent coronary artery with TIMI III flow, using the Thrombolysis in Myocardial Infarction (TIMI) grading for coronary blood flow. Conventionally, angiographic no-reflow is indicated by ≤TIMI flow II. However, using myocardial contrast echocardiography to detect no-reflow in PPCI patients, Ito et al., (1996) reported that 100% of patients with TIMI II flow displayed evidence of MVO as detected by contrast echocardiography. They also found that 16% of patients with TIMI III flow demonstrated MVO, confirming that a patent coronary artery does not necessarily equate to effective myocardial perfusion.

Further methods of classification such as the TIMI frame count, the myocardial blush grade, and the TIMI myocardial perfusion grade have been introduced to better recognize and assess impaired myocardial perfusion. Studies have validated the myocardial blush grade and the TIMI myocardial perfusion grade as indicators of no-reflow and have linked the presence of impaired myocardial perfusion with adverse effects on myocardial infarct size, LV ejection fraction and clinical outcomes.

The resolution of ST-segment elevation and early T-wave inversion following restoration of blood flow in the infarct-related coronary artery following PPCI is suggestive of successful myocardial perfusion. Conversely, persistent ST-elevation following PCI may indicate coronary no-reflow associated with adverse clinical outcomes (Claeys et al., 1999), and so the 12-lead ECG may provide initial evidence of the no-reflow phenomenon.

Using a Doppler guidewire to obtain the coronary flow velocity profile following PPCI, the presence of coronary no-reflow may be represented by systolic flow reversal, reduced anterograde systolic flow and forward diastolic flow with a rapid deceleration slope, a flow pattern which impedes coronary blood flow and is associated with TIMI II flow and impaired LV ejection fraction (Iwakura et al., 1996; Akasaka et al., 2000). In the presence of coronary microemboli in the distal coronary circulation the flow profile is characterized by slow forward flow and an increase in the diastolic to systolic flow ratio due to augmented coronary resistance (Yamamoto et al., 2002).

5.3.2 **Non-invasive imaging to detect MVO**

With recent advances in non-invasive cardiac imaging it is now possible to detect and visualize the phenomenon of microvascular obstruction, the cause of coronary no-reflow, in patients following primary PCI. The presence of a myocardial perfusion defect can be detected using either myocardial perfusion nuclear scanning, myocardial contrast echocardiography or contrast-enhanced cardiac MRI.

Myocardial Contrast Echocardiography

Gas-filled microbubbles similar in size to red blood cells, which remain within the intravascular compartment, are injected intravenously as a constant infusion to achieve a steady state level. These microbubbles are able to traverse the pulmonary circulation. After 2–3 minutes the bubbles appear in the LV cavity and the myocardium blood pool, where they increase signal intensity. A high-energy ultrasound pulse is then used to destroy the microbubbles and the rate of myocardial *re-uptake* of microbubbles is then used to determine myocardial perfusion. Due to microvascular obstruction, in areas of no-reflow the myocardial uptake of microbubbles is delayed and the myocardium appears devoid of any acoustic signal (Kaul 2006). Pre-clinical studies have recently reported that it is now possible to conjugate microbubbles with antibodies or ligands which bind to and target activated adhesion molecules on the vascular endothelium, enabling the visualisation of areas of myocardial inflammation and other pathophysiological processes that contribute to MVO (Kaufmann & Lindner, 2007).

Myocardial Perfusion Nuclear Scanning

Myocardial perfusion nuclear scanning can also be used to detect MVO in patients recently recanalised following an AMI. Clinical studies using ^{99m}Tc tetrofosmin single photon emission computed tomographic (SPECT) imaging have demonstrated that the absent uptake of tracer in the presence of a patent infarct-related coronary artery indicates a myocardial perfusion defect at the level of the microvasculature (Kondo *et al.*, 1998).

Gadolinium-enhanced cardiac MRI

Gadolinium (Gd)-enhanced cardiac MRI can be used to detect both microvascular obstruction (MVO) and delineate infarcted myocardium in patients with reperfused STEMI. Initial clinical studies from the mid-1990's first reported the application of contrast-enhanced cardiac MRI for detecting MVO in reperfused AMI patients (Lima *et al.*, 1995; Wu *et al.*, 1998; Rochitte *et al.*, 1998). Following the injection of Gd, the early myocardial uptake (first-pass 2–3 min) of the contrast agent (termed 'wash-in') signifies normally perfused myocardium. In the presence of MVO, the 'wash-in' of Gd is delayed leaving an area of myocardium devoid of contrast, which corresponds to the region of MVO (see Figure 5.1). However, the size of this region reduces with

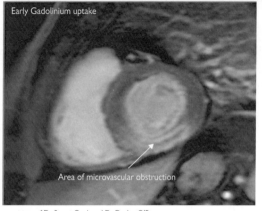

Figure 5.1 Microvascular obstruction detected by a zone lacking early gadolinium uptake on cardiac MRI in patient with a PCI reperfused inferior STEMI

Early Gadolinium uptake

Area of microvascular obstruction

Image courtesy of Dr Stuart Cook and Dr Declan O'Regan

time as contrast slowly penetrates this area. Subsequent delayed imaging (12–15 min) depicts 'wash-out' of the contrast agent but Gd remains in the infarcted myocardium due to cardiomyocyte necrosis, leaving a core of hypo-enhancement which also corresponds to the area of MVO. Using this technique the extent of MVO has been demonstrated to increase over the first 48 hours of reperfusion, confirming its description as a form of myocardial reperfusion injury (Rochitte et al., 1998).

5.4 Treatment of Coronary No-Reflow

5.4.1 Mechanical interventions

Ischaemic postconditioning

Ischaemic postconditioning (IPost) represents the most promising of the mechanical interventions for preventing coronary no-reflow in reperfused STEMI patients (Tsang et al., 2004; Vinten-Johansen et al., 2007). By interrupting myocardial reperfusion with several short-lived episodes of myocardial ischaemia, this mechanical intervention has been demonstrated to improve myocardial reperfusion in STEMI patients undergoing PCI, as evidenced by improved myocardial blush grade (Staat et al., 2005), better ST-segment resolution (Laskey 2005), faster coronary frame TIMI count (Ma et al., 2006), increased coronary flow velocity reserve (Laskey 2005), improved endothelial function (Ma *et al.*, 2006), augmented wall motion score index (Ma *et al.*, 2006), and reduced malondialdehyde levels (a non-specific measure of oxidative stress). Furthermore, IPost has been reported to reduce myocardial infarct size in reperfused STEMI patients (see Chapter 11).

Distal protection and Thrombectomy

Distal embolization of atheroma and thrombus occurs in 9–15% of primary PCI cases, and is associated with worse clinical outcomes. It may contribute to the phenomenon of no-reflow by causing coronary microembolization, which is a feature of MVO (van Gaal & Banning, 2007). Distal protection devices (which prevent the embolization of thrombus and plaque) and thrombectomy (devices for aspirating thrombus) are clearly beneficial in patients undergoing PCI of vein graft occlusions and in patients receiving rotational atherectomy (van Gaal & Banning, 2007), but the large multi-centred AIMI (Ali *et al.*, 2006) and EMERALD (Stone *et al.*, 2005) clinical trials examining this intervention in primary PCI patients have failed to demonstrate any beneficial effects on myocardial reperfusion, infarct size or on the clinical outcomes of death or re-infarction (Kunadian *et al.*, 2007).

5.4.2 Pharmacological interventions

Adenosine

Adenosine is an endogenous purine nucleoside which is generated during myocardial ischaemia. It has the ability to act as a powerful endogenous vascular protectant through several mechanisms including: the inhibition of neutrophil activation and neutrophil-vascular interactions; protecting endothelial function; and inducing coronary vasodilatation.

Clinical studies of primary PCI patients have demonstrated beneficial effects of intracoronary adenosine (administered as bolus of about 70 mcg) in terms of less coronary no-reflow (Assali *et al.*, 2000). The beneficial effects of intracoronary adenosine when used in conjunction with other pharmacological agents such as nitroprusside, nicorandil have also been studied and shown to produce additive effects.

Calcium Channel Blockers

Intracoronary infusions of calcium channel blockers have been given to target the microvascular vasoconstriction that contributes to coronary reflow in patients undergoing primary PCI. Intracoronary verapamil (using a bolus of 1 mg) as adjunctive therapy improved coronary blood flow as evidence by TIMI flow, TIMI frame count, and TIMI perfusion grade, reduced no-reflow (assessed by myocardial contrast echocardiography), improved myocardial perfusion (assessed by SPECT), increased the wall motion score index, and preserved LV systolic function (Werner *et al.*, 2002; Hang *et al.*, 2005).

K_{ATP} Channel Opening

Preclinical studies have implicated the ATP-dependent potassium channel (mK_{ATP}) as a critical mediator of endogenous cardioprotection (Yellon & Downey, 2003). However, the reports examining the beneficial effects of pharmacologically opening the mK_{ATP} at the onset of myocardial reperfusion have been inconclusive. Nicorandil, which is a purported opener of this channel, has been investigated as adjunctive therapy to PPCI in several clinical studies, although it can also act as a nitric oxide donor. A number of clinical studies have reported beneficial effects of intravenous nicorandil (about 10 mg over 24 hrs) administered as adjunctive therapy to primary PCI in terms of less coronary no-reflow, better ST-segment resolution, higher TIMI frame-counts, and improved wall-motion score index (Ito et al., 1999; Ono et al., 2004). Unfortunately, the recent 545 patient J-WIND-KATP (Japan-Working groups of acute myocardial infarction for the reduction of Necrotic Damage) trial failed to demonstrate any beneficial effects of nicorandil as adjunctive therapy to primary PCI, on myocardial infarct size, LV ejection fraction or clinical outcomes (Kitakaze et al., 2007).

Other antioxidant agents such as edaravone (Tsujita et al., 2006) have been examined as adjuvants to PPCI in small proof-of-concept clinical trials and have reported beneficial effects on no-reflow, LV ejection fraction, infarct size and clinical outcomes. Whether these findings extrapolate to an improvement in meaningful long-term clinical outcomes remains to be determined. Novel antioxidant reperfusion therapies under investigation include melatonin in the MARIA (Melatonin Adjunct in the acute myocaRdial Infarction treated with Angioplasty) trial (Dominguez-Rodriguez et al., 2007).

5.5 Conclusions

The inability to perfuse a previously ischaemic myocardium on restoring coronary blood flow in the infarct-related coronary artery characterizes the coronary 'no-reflow' phenomenon, the cause of which is obstruction at the level of the microvasculature. Microvascular obstruction occurs in 30–60% of reperfused STEMI patients and is associated with larger infarct sizes, poor LV ejection fraction, adverse LV remodelling and worse clinical outcomes. Its presence can be detected in the catheter laboratory by impeded coronary artery flow, poor ST-segment resolution and impaired myocardial perfusion. Its presence can also be detected using non-invasive imaging modalities such as nuclear myocardial perfusion scanning, myocardial contrast echocardiography and contrast-enhanced cardiac MRI as a myocardial perfusion defect. Current therapeutic strategies include intracoronary vasodilators such as adenosine, calcium-channel blockers, and nitrates.

Newer treatment strategies are required to prevent and reduce this form of myocardial reperfusion injury so that clinical outcomes in STEMI patients may be improved.

Key references

Akasaka, T., Yoshida, K., Kawamoto, T., *et al.*, (2000). Relation of phasic coronary flow velocity characteristics with TIMI perfusion grade and myocardial recovery after primary percutaneous transluminal coronary angioplasty and rescue stenting. *Circulation*, **101**: 2361–2367.

Ali A, Cox D, Dib N., *et al.*, (2006). Rheolytic thrombectomy with percutaneous coronary intervention for infarct size reduction in acute myocardial infarction: 30-day results from a multicenter randomized study. *J Am Coll Cardiol*, **48**: 244–252.

Assali, A.R., Sdringola, S., Ghani, M., *et al.*, (2000). Intracoronary adenosine administered during percutaneous intervention in acute myocardial infarction and reduction in the incidence of 'no reflow' phenomenon. *Catheter Cardiovasc Interv*, **51**: 27–31.

Claeys, M.J., Bosmans, J., Veenstra, L., *et al.*, (1999). Determinants and prognostic implications of persistent ST-segment elevation after primary angioplasty for acute myocardial infarction: importance of microvascular reperfusion injury on clinical outcome. *Circulation*, **99**: 1972–1977.

De Luca, G., 't Hof, A.W., de Boer, M.J., *et al.*, (2004). Impaired myocardial perfusion is a major explanation of the poor outcome observed in patients undergoing primary angioplasty for ST-segment-elevation myocardial infarction and signs of heart failure. *Circulation*, **109**: 958–961.

Dominguez-Rodriguez, A., Abreu-Gonzalez, P., Garcia-Gonzalez, M., *et al.*, (2007). A unicenter, randomized, double-blind, parallel-group, placebo-controlled study of Melatonin as an Adjunct in patients with acute myocaRdial Infarction undergoing primary Angioplasty The Melatonin Adjunct in the acute myocaRdial Infarction treated with Angioplasty (MARIA) trial: study design and rationale. *Contemp Clin Trials*, **28**: 532–539.

Hang, C.L., Wang, C.P., Yip, H.K., *et al.*, (2005). Early administration of intracoronary verapamil improves myocardial perfusion during percutaneous coronary interventions for acute myocardial infarction. *Chest*, **128**: 2593–2598.

Ito, H. (2006). No-reflow phenomenon and prognosis in patients with acute myocardial infarction. *Nat Clin Pract Cardiovasc Med*, **3**: 499–506.

Ito, H., Okamura, A., Iwakura, K., *et al.*, (1996). Myocardial perfusion patterns related to thrombolysis in myocardial infarction perfusion grades after coronary angioplasty in patients with acute anterior wall myocardial infarction. *Circulation*, **93**: 1993–1999.

Ito, H., Taniyama, Y., Iwakura, K., *et al.*, (1999). Intravenous nicorandil can preserve microvascular integrity and myocardial viability in patients with reperfused anterior wall myocardial infarction. *J Am Coll Cardiol*, **33**: 654–660.

Iwakura, K., Ito, H., Kawano S., *et al.*, (2001). Predictive factors for development of the no-reflow phenomenon in patients with reperfused anterior wall acute myocardial infarction. *J Am Coll Cardiol*, **38**: 472–477.

Iwakura, K., Ito, H., Takiuchi, S., Fujii, K., and Minamino, T. (1996). Alternation in the coronary blood flow velocity pattern in patients with no reflow and reperfused acute myocardial infarction. *Circulation*, **94**: 1269–1275.

Kaufmann, B.A., Lindner, J.R. (2007). Molecular imaging with targeted contrast ultrasound. *Curr Opin Biotechnol*, **18**: 11–16.

Kaul S. (2006). Evaluating the 'no reflow' phenomenon with myocardial contrast echocardiography. *Basic Res Cardiol*, **101**: 391–399.

Kitakaze, M., Asakura, M., Kim, J., *et al.*, (2007). Human atrial natriuretic peptide and nicorandil as adjuncts to reperfusion treatment for acute myocardial infarction (J-WIND): two randomized trials. *Lancet*, **370**: 1483–1493.

Kloner, R.A., Ganote, C.E., Jennings, R.B. (1974). The 'no-reflow' phenomenon after temporary coronary occlusion in the dog. *J Clin Invest*, **54**: 1496–1508.

Kondo, M., Nakano, A., Saito, D., Shimono, Y. (1998). Assessment of 'microvascular no-reflow phenomenon' using technetium-99m macro-aggregated albumin scintigraphy in patients with acute myocardial infarction. *J Am Coll Cardiol*, **32**: 898–903.

Krug, A., Du Mesnil, D.R., Korb, G. (1966). Blood supply of the myocardium after temporary coronary occlusion. *Circ Res*, **19**: 57–62.

Kunadian, B., Dunning, J., Vijayalakshmi, K., *et al.*, (2007). Meta-analysis of randomized trials comparing anti-embolic devices with standard PCI for improving myocardial reperfusion in patients with acute myocardial infarction. *Catheter Cardiovasc Interv*, **69**: 488–496.

Laskey, W.K. (2005). Brief repetitive balloon occlusions enhance reperfusion during percutaneous coronary intervention for acute myocardial infarction: a pilot study. *Catheter Cardiovasc Interv*, **65**: 361–367.

Lima, J.A., Judd, R.M., Bazille, A., *et al.*, (1995). Regional heterogeneity of human myocardial infarcts demonstrated by contrast-enhanced MRI. Potential mechanisms. *Circulation*, **92**: 1117–1125.

Ma, X., Zhang, X., Li, C., Luo, M. (2006). Effect of Postconditioning on Coronary Blood Flow Velocity and Endothelial Function and LV Recovery After Myocardial Infarction. *J Interv Cardiol*, **19**: 367–375.

Ono, H., Osanai, T., Ishizaka, H., *et al.*, (2004). Nicorandil improves cardiac function and clinical outcome in patients with acute myocardial infarction undergoing primary percutaneous coronary intervention: role of inhibitory effect on reactive oxygen species formation. *Am Heart J*, **148**: E15.

Rochitte, C.E., Lima, J.A., Bluemke, D.A., *et al.*, (1998). Magnitude and time course of microvascular obstruction and tissue injury after acute myocardial infarction. *Circulation*, **98**: 1006–1014.

Staat, P., Rioufol, G., Piot, C., *et al.*, (2005). Postconditioning the human heart. *Circulation*, **112**: 2143–2148.

Stone, G.W., Webb, J., Cox, D.A., et al., (2005). Distal microcirculatory protection during percutaneous coronary intervention in acute ST-segment elevation myocardial infarction: a randomized controlled trial. *JAMA*, **293**: 1063–1072.

Tsang, A., Hausenloy, D.J., Mocanu, M.M., Yellon D.M. (2004). Postconditioning: a form of 'modified reperfusion' protects the myocardium by activating the phosphatidylinositol 3-kinase-Akt pathway. *Circ Res*, **95**: 230–232.

Tsujita, K., Shimomura, H., Kaikita, K., et al., (2006). Long-term efficacy of edaravone in patients with acute myocardial infarction. *Circ J*, **70**: 832–837.

van Gaal, W.J., Banning A.P. (2007). Percutaneous coronary intervention and the no-reflow phenomenon. *Expert Rev Cardiovasc Ther*, **5**: 715–731.

Vinten-Johansen J. (2007). Postconditioning: a mechanical maneuver that triggers biological and molecular cardioprotective responses to reperfusion. *Heart Fail Rev*, **12**: 235–244.

Werner, G.S., Lang, K., Kuehnert, H., Figulla, H.R. (2002). Intracoronary verapamil for reversal of no-reflow during coronary angioplasty for acute myocardial infarction. *Catheter Cardiovasc Interv*, **57**: 444–451.

Wu, K.C., Zerhouni, E.A., Judd, R.M., et al., (1998). Prognostic significance of microvascular obstruction by magnetic resonance imaging in patients with acute myocardial infarction. *Circulation*, **97**: 765–772.

Yamamoto, K., Ito, H., Iwakura, K., et al., (2002). Two different coronary blood flow velocity patterns in thrombolysis in myocardial infarction flow grade 2 in acute myocardial infarction: insight into mechanisms of microvascular dysfunction. *J Am Coll Cardiol*, **40**: 1755–1760.

Yellon, D.M., Downey J.M. (2003). Preconditioning the myocardium: from cellular physiology to clinical cardiology. *Physiol Rev*, **83**: 1113–1151.

Chapter 6

Optimal Medical Therapy Post-AMI

Lionel Opie

Key points

- The management of an acute myocardial infarction can be divided into four phases: (a) The initial acute ischaemia causes severe prolonged chest pain when the patient is rushed to a Coronary or Intensive Care Unit; (b) Within the next few hours as ischaemia changes into infarction, the aim at this step is to restore blood flow in the occluded artery by thrombolysis or by percutaneous coronary intervention (PCI); (c) Next, the infarct is established and the left ventricle undergoes early remodeling; (d) Finally, follows the post-AMI post-hospital phase when continued left ventricular remodeling takes place

- The therapeutic management of each of these steps can be optimized using appropriate medical therapy including antiplatelet and antithrombotic therapy, beta-blockers, ACE-inhibitors and angiotensin receptor blockers, lipid-lowering drugs, aldosterone antagonists, omega-3 fatty acids and so on.

6.1 Introduction

Myocardial infarction is, by definition, a process whereby cells undergo cell death and, in clinical terms, is a syndrome of coronary occlusion causing severe chest pain with characteristic ST-segment elevation (STEMI) on the ECG, and elevated blood levels of enzymes of cardiac origin such as troponin. Major cell death may take about 3 hours of severe ischaemia (lack of blood flow) to develop, giving a 'golden gap' for intervention by reperfusion (Gersh *et al.*, 2005). This chapter will focus on four different phases of the therapeutic care of AMI (Figure 6.1): (1) The initial acute ischaemia causes severe prolonged chest pain when the patient is rushed to a Coronary or Intensive Care Unit; relief of chest pain and antiplatelet therapy by aspirin and/or clopidogrel are all crucial; (2) Within the next few hours as ischaemia changes into infarction, the aim is to restore blood flow in the occluded artery by early reperfusion using thrombolysis or by percutaneous coronary intervention (PCI) covered by inhibitors of the glycoprotein IIb/IIIa platelet receptors; control of reperfusion injury by insulin-glucose is under test, while the patient may require drugs that interrupt the adverse metabolic-hormonal response such as beta-blockers and renin-angiotensin inhibitors; (3) Next, as the infarct is established, the left ventricle undergoes early remodelling, while the patient is haemodynamically stable and beta-blockers and renin-angiotensin inhibitors are often given; and (4) Finally follows the post-AMI post-hospital phase when continued left ventricular remodelling, started during the acute phase of AMI, may proceed to increasing left ventricular failure which calls for diuretics and (if not yet given) beta-blockers and renin-angiotensin inhibitors. However, in a minority with small or aborted infarcts, excellent effort tolerance is possible. Other medications such as aldosterone antagonists, statins and omega fish oils, may now be added to the therapy.

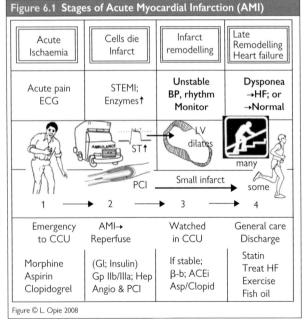

Figure 6.1 Stages of Acute Myocardial Infarction (AMI)

Acute Ischaemia	Cells die Infarct	Infarct remodelling	Late Remodelling Heart failure
Acute pain ECG	STEMI; Enzymes↑	**Unstable BP, rhythm Monitor**	**Dysponea →HF; or →Normal**
1	2	3	4
Emergency to CCU	AMI→ Reperfuse	Watched in CCU	General care Discharge
Morphine Aspirin Clopidogrel	(GI; Insulin) Gp IIb/IIIa; Hep Angio & PCI	If stable; β-b; ACEi Asp/Clopid	Statin Treat HF Exercise Fish oil

Figure © L. Opie 2008

In phase 1 of acute myocardial infarction (AMI), the patient has acute prolonged chest pain and requires morphine to relieve pain, and platelet inhibition by aspirin and clopidogrel (Asp/clopid) while being transported to a Coronary Care Unit (CCU). In phase 2, the ideal is administration of platelet receptor blockers (Gp IIb/IIIa) and anti-coagulants (Hep, heparin; or low molecular weight heparin) followed by coronary angiography (angio) and reperfusion by percutaneous coronary intervention (PCI). In phase 3, the left ventricle remodels and often dilates, while the patient is monitored and evaluated for therapy by beta-blockers (β-b) and angiotensin converting enzyme inhibitors (ACEi). In phase 4, the patient has left the CCU and is now ready for discharge; therapy often includes a statin, a diuretic if needed for heart failure, fish-oil capsules to counter post-infarct sudden death, and exercise instructions. Note the major effect of infarct size on exercise capacity.

6.1.1 Therapeutic challenges

This chapter examines the following aspects in greater detail. Can early phase metabolic therapy lessen the extent of cell necrosis and alter the acute general hormonal and metabolic response that results in adverse mobilisation of free fatty acids (FFA) and the inhibition of beneficial glucose metabolism? Should beta-blockade be given very early? As ischaemic cells die, ventricular remodelling with risk of heart failure sets in – can this process be limited by inhibitors of the renin-angiotensin-aldosterone (RAAS) system? Finally, what is optimal chronic post-AMI therapy? Beta-blockade, ACE-inhibitors and statins make a good preventative trio.

6.2 Early phase metabolic intervention for AMI

Metabolically, the two major features of early phase AMI are:

1. an acute general metabolic reaction, resulting in stress-mediated catecholamine mobilization which increases levels of blood free fatty acids (FFA) (Vetter et al., 1974) and promotes glucose intolerance; and

2. the local myocardial lesion in which the critical feature is lack of blood flow (ischaemia) which if sufficiently prolonged causes cell death by necrosis. In response to such severe hypoxia, the cell has a self-regulating defence mechanism whereby glycolysis is increased to provide anaerobic ATP, even in the absence of oxygen and despite the low blood flow. Furthermore, emergency pro-survival kinase signalling systems are activated, including those that are stimulated by insulin (Hausenloy & Yellon, 2006). These self-protective mechanisms are countered by the adverse effects

of high blood free fatty acids, as shown in classic studies by Michael Oliver (Oliver et al., 1968). He argued that these fatty acids were damaging heart cell membranes by demanding excess oxygen. Logically, the administration of glucose and insulin (the 'glucose hypothesis') (Opie, 1970) should counter FFA-mediated damage (de Leiris et al., 1975) and promote the activity of the prosurvival kinases (Hausenloy & Yellon, 2006).

Therefore, it seems reasonable to postulate a metabolic approach to cardiac protection whereby the effects of glucose and insulin are 'good' and those of catecholamines and free fatty acids are 'bad'. This metabolic approach to myocardial infarction is, strangely enough, still under test even so many years after Sodi-Pallares first wrote about glucose-insulin-potassium (GIK) in 1962. Most of the outcome studies with GIK have failed to study the first few hours early after the onset of AMI when plasma catecholamines and FFA are highest (Chaudhuri et al., 2007) or during the reperfusion period when insulin should be active in reducing reperfusion damage (Yellon & Hausenloy, 2007). Preliminary work with ischaemic postconditioning in patients suggests that with modern early primary PCI, perhaps one-third of the reperfused cells die instead of surviving (Staat et al., 2005).

6.2.1 Strict glucose control?

Acute myocardial infarction (AMI) is a diabetogenic disease as it may precipitate diabetes, both in the acute stage and several years later (Opie, 2007). Increased plasma glucose is associated with a worse prognosis in AMI, so it would be logical to reduce the blood glucose value. Indeed, in the DIGAMI trial on diabetic patients with AMI, infusions of insulin (covered by glucose to avoid hypoglycaemia) and continued insulin treatment after discharge from hospital for three months, reduced mortality in patients with AMI (Malmberg et al., 1995). However, extrapolating from experiences in Medical Intensive Care Units (ICUs) (Van den Berghe et al., 2006), the danger of an insulin-based approach aimed at reducing the blood glucose to eugly-caemia is hypoglycaemia, raising the risk of death and partially coun-tering the overall benefits of glucose reduction. Modified low dose GIK (10% dextrose with KCl 40 mmol at 60 ml/h with regular human insulin at 2.5 units/h) was able to lower FFA from toxic levels in controls (1.6 mmol/l) to approximately 1.0 mmol/l, within the physio-logical albumin-binding range (Chaudhuri et al., 2007). In the large INTENSIVE trial, intensive insulin therapy is being tested against sliding scale insulin with infarct size as the end-point, the hypothesis being that insulin has anti-inflammatory properties that could thereby reduce infarct size.

Another potential mechanism of benefit is unrelated to the ambient blood glucose or to any effects on glycaemia, and tests the potential therapeutic role of insulin when on board at the time of reperfusion, where extensive animal work strongly suggests that reperfusion damage can be limited by the kinase pathways stimulated by several agents including insulin given at that time (Yellon & Opie, 2006). This possibility will be indirectly tested in the ongoing NIH-supported IMMEDIATE study starting glucose-insulin-potassium (GIK) in the ambulance, and continuing in the hospital Emergency Room beyond the time of reperfusion therapy. This study may provide conclusive data regarding the efficacy of GIK therapy. Any benefit could be explained by either a metabolic effect on the infarcting myocardium by promoting glucose metabolism and inhibiting that of FFA or by insulin-mediated decreased reperfusion injury or by both mechanisms. In the future, GLP-1 or exenatide, agents acting on the incretin system, may be the preferred glycaemia lowering agents because they avoid hypoglycaemia, while promoting endogenous insulin secretion. These are trials that must still be undertaken.

6.3 Beta-blockers

In previous times when serious ventricular arrhythmias, including fibrillation, often brought early fatality even in CCUs, early beta-blockade was commonly undertaken. The rationale was that AMI stimulated the adrenergic system which, in turn, elevated myocardial tissue cyclic AMP, a strong pro-arrhythmic agent acting by increased calcium loading and oscillations (Lubbe et al., 1992). In one clinical study (Norris et al., 1984), intravenous propranolol given during early phase AMI reduced ventricular fibrillation. However, with the advent of increased access to CCUs and better arrhythmia monitoring, early death by ventricular fibrillation has become an unusual event. In the only available study in which early beta-blockade was routinely given intravenously to patients receiving thrombolytic therapy, ventricular fibrillation was indeed reduced as predicted but there were excess deaths from cardiogenic shock and hypotension (Chen et al., 2005). Whereas the excess of cardiogenic shock occurred mainly in the first day after admission, reduced reinfarction and ventricular fibrillation emerged more gradually. The major lesson to emerge was that the routine early intravenous beta-blockade was potentially harmful, particularly in those who were haemodynamically unstable. A separate issue is whether the later administration of beta-blockade, when haemodynamic stability had been attained, would be more beneficial as suggested by the same trial (Chen et al., 2005).

In the only study comparing early intravenous and later oral beta-blockade, immediate intravenous beta-blockade given within two hours of starting reperfusion was compared with delayed oral beta-blockade, started on the sixth day (Roberts et al., 1991). Although early intravenous beta-blockade reduced early myocardial ischaemia and reinfarction in the first week, over one year there was no difference. Emerging from these and other conflicting studies, the current practice is to start beta-blockade (if no contraindications) within the first few days of hospitalization once the patient is haemodynamically stable and to consider early urgent beta-blockade for compelling indications such as severe hypertension or tachycardias. Although this recommendation is standard in guidelines, there appear to be no hard data to suggest exactly when and how beta-blockade should be initiated.

A number of observational studies suggest that beta-blockade could be given with benefit to cover primary percutaneous intervention (PPCI), when the metabolic benefit of lowering plasma FFA should theoretically add to that of blood-flow induced restoration of tissue glycolysis that had been inhibited during the period of severe ischaemia. However, there are no prospective studies as required for proof of concept. On the other hand, there are compelling data indicating that every post-infarct patient should be considered for beta-blockade to help to prevent development of heart failure and to reduce sudden death. Thus almost all patients with AMI should be receiving beta-blockade, unless contraindicated, before the end of their hospitalisation for AMI.

6.4 ACE inhibitors/ARB's

As AMI is accompanied by activation of the renin-angiotensin-aldosterone system (RAAS), and both angiotensin and aldosterone have numerous potentially deleterious effects that include the promotion of adverse myocardial remodelling, it is logical to consider the use of angiotensin converting enzyme (ACE) inhibitors, angiotensin receptor blockers (ARBs) and aldosterone antagonists. There are two current controversies. First, should acute RAS inhibition be given only to those patients who are more acutely ill in the first few days of AMI or should this type of therapy be given to all patients? In practice many clinicians opt not to use ACE-inhibitors in patients who are otherwise very well controlled from the hemodynamic and lipid and blood pressure points of view. Another controversy relates to the follow up period after myocardial infarction. If ACE-inhibitors slow the progress of coronary disease as shown by two large prospective studies, namely HOPE and EUROPA, then surely all post-AMI patients should receive an ACE-inhibitor? Yet in one other study, PEACE, on very well treated patients with stable coronary disease, there was absolutely no effect of an ACE-inhibitor, not even in those with a prior AMI (Braunwald et al., 2004). Although when all three studies are taken together, there are dominant beneficial effects

(Dagenais *et al.*, 2006), the two positive studies were long term prophylactic on high-risk patients (HOPE and EUROPA), while PEACE was on post-infarct patients. One postulate is that post-infarct ACE-inhibition was ineffective in PEACE because the patients were already very well treated by revascularization (in 72%), beta- or calcium-blocker therapy (almost all) and lipid-lowering (70%). If, however, the patient has overt left ventricular failure or left ventricular dysfunction in AMI, then ACE-inhibitors are standard therapy. Regarding their early use within 24 hours of the onset of AMI, Dr Marc Pfeffer and I (Opie & Pfeffer, 2008), favour a selective policy which is to give ACE-inhibitors specifically to all high risk patients, namely diabetics, those with anterior infarct or with tachycardia or with LV failure. Logically, the sicker the patient, the greater the degree of the renin-angiotensin system activation and the better the expected result. Thus in those with large infarcts or with diabetes, ACE-inhibitors give a striking 26% reduction in mortality.

6.5 **ARBs and heart failure**

ARBs have been tested in an era when ACE-inhibitors were already the established therapy of choice for heart failure. Had the ARBs come earlier, they would probably have been first choice. Taking together the results of several large trials such as Val-HeFT, CHARM and VALIANT, the ARBs in the specific doses used are not inferior to ACE-inhibitors, whether the basic problem is heart failure or post-infarct protection (Opie and Pfeffer, 2008). Thus the ARB valsartan was equivalent to captopril in reducing death and adverse cardiovascular outcomes, with decreased cough, rash and taste disturbances (VALIANT trial). The downside was increased hypotension and renal problems.

6.6 **Aldosterone antagonists**

Regarding aldosterone, recent clinical studies show that increased aldosterone levels in AMI are associated with a worse clinical outcome. Classically, increased aldosterone secretion is the termination of the RAAS. Experimentally, there are substantial data to show that aldosterone promotes myocardial fibrosis. Extrapolation from experience in hypertension studies suggest that when there is sodium-retention as in AMI with heart failure, the normal sodium-induced suppression of aldosterone may fail (Pratt, 2008). Aldosterone levels are associated with adverse clinical outcomes including mortality in ST-elevation MI (Beygui *et al.*, 2006). Specifically, aldosterone has adverse vascular effects including inhibition of release of nitric oxide, and an increased response to vasoconstrictor doses of angiotensin-I in human heart failure (Farquharson & Struthers, 2000). From these points of view, therapy with an aldosterone blocker such as spironolactone or eplerenone, becomes potentially desirable for those with AMI, whatever the stage, but especially for patients with LV dysfunction. The combination of these drugs with ACE-inhibitors or ARBs requires special care in monitoring serum potassium, which could rapidly rise to abnormal levels with threat of potentially fatal cardiac arrhythmias.

6.7 Lipid-lowering therapy

The standard lipid lowering agents are the statins, which act to inhibit the formation of low density lipoprotein cholesterol (LDL-C) in the liver, thereby decreasing circulating LDL-cholesterol. Epidemiologically, there is a straight-line relationship between the reduction in the LDL-C level and the reduction by statins of coronary heart disease events (Fisher, 2004). Meta-analyses of a very large number of patients suggests that anyone with vascular disease including myocardial infarction should automatically be given a statin, irrespective of the initial blood lipid levels. Furthermore, LDL-C levels change spontaneously within the first few weeks after myocardial infarction, so there is little justification for watchful waiting to decide whether or not to give a statin. Rather, the statin should be started during the hospital stay, after the acute phase of AMI so the patient leaves hospital with a statin. Because of the benefit of statins and their possible anti-inflammatory and non-lipid (pleiotropic) effects, many physicians choose to start statin therapy soon after the admission of the patient to the CCU, say within the first few days. However the trial data are from two major studies giving high-dose statins after acute coronary syndromes, 33–40% with STEMI, the one started within 5 days of the event and the other 10 days (Murphy et al., 2007). One death was prevented by treating 95 patients with high-dose statin therapy for two years. What now needs translation into clinical practice is the finding that statins given experimentally at the time of reperfusion decrease reperfusion-induced infarction, another pleiotropic effect (Mensah et al., 2005).

6.8 Omega-3 polyunsaturated fatty acids and fish oils

In the very important GISSI-Prevenzione study, in the post-infarct period a large number of post-AMI patients were randomized to either n-3 polyunsaturated fatty acids (PUFAs, 1 gram daily) capsules or to placebo (Marchioli et al., 2002). Those who received the n-3 PUFAs had a lessened sudden death and decreased mortality. These findings are supported by epidemiological studies showing that fish consumption is inversely related to fatal coronary heart disease (He *et al.*, 2004). Of note, the traditional Mediterranean diet is high in omega-3 fatty acids and also associated with lower rates of myocardial infarction. The mechanism concerned has not been fully clarified, but several laboratory studies show that omega-3 oils have antiarrhythmic properties (Den Ruijter *et al.*, 2008), potentially by improving the myocardial membrane structure. Thus, the justification for an omega-3 rich diet or omega-3 capsules after myocardial infarction is strong.

6.9 Summary

Acute myocardial infarction (AMI) can arbitrarily be divided into four phases. In the first, the patient has acute prolonged chest pain and requires morphine to relieve pain, and platelet inhibition by aspirin and/or clopidogrel while being transported to the nearest Coronary Care Unit (CCU). Next, in phase two the aim is to reopen the occluded artery by thrombolysis or percutaneous coronary intervention (PCI) under cover of heparin while antiplatelet therapy is intensified (Gp IIb/IIIa receptor blockers). In the third phase, the left ventricle remodels and often dilates, while the patient is monitored and evaluated for therapy by beta-blockers, ACE-inhibitors or ARBs and/or aldosterone blockers. In the fourth phase, discharge medications usually include aspirin/clopidogrel, beta-blockers, ACE-inhibitors or ARBs, statins, diuretics as needed for heart failure, fish-oil capsules to counter post-infarct sudden death, and exercise instructions. Note the major effect of infarct size on exercise capacity.

Key references

Beygui, F., Collet, JP., Benoliel, J.J., *et al.*, (2006). High plasma aldosterone levels on admission are associated with death in patients presenting with acute ST-elevation myocardial infarction. *Circulation*, **114**: 2604–2610.

Braunwald, E., Domanski, M.J., Fowler, S.E., *et al.*, (2004). Angiotensin-converting-enzyme inhibition in stable coronary artery disease. *N Engl J Med*, **351**: 2058–2068.

Chaudhuri, A., Janicke, D., Wilson, M., *et al.*, (2007). Effect of modified glucose-insulin-potassium on free fatty acids, matrix metalloproteinase, and myoglobin in ST-elevation myocardial infarction. *Am J Cardiol*, **100**: 1614–1618.

Chen, Z.M., Pan, H.C., Chen, Y.P., *et al.*, (2005). Early intravenous then oral metoprolol in 45,852 patients with acute myocardial infarction: randomized placebo-controlled trial. *Lancet*, **366**: 1622–1632.

Dagenais, G.R., Pogue, J., Fox, K., *et al.*, (2006). Angiotensin-converting-enzyme inhibitors in stable vascular disease without left ventricular systolic dysfunction or heart failure: a combined analysis of three trials. *Lancet*, **368**: 581–588.

de Leiris, J., Opie, L.H., Lubbe, W.F. (1975). Effects of free fatty acid and glucose on enzyme release in experimental myocardial infarction. *Nature*, **253**: 746–747.

Den Ruijter, H.M., Berecki, G., Verkerk, A.O., *et al.,* (2008). Acute administration of fish oil inhibits triggered activity in isolated myocytes from rabbits and patients with heart failure. *Circulation*, **117**: 536–544.

Farquharson, C.A.J., Struthers, A.D. (2000). Spironolactone increases nitric oxide bioactivity, improves endothelial vasodilator dysfunction, and suppresses vascular angiotensin I/angiotensin II conversion in patients with chronic heart failure. *Circulation*, **101**: 594–597.

Fisher, M. (2004). Diabetes and atherogenesis. *Heart*, **90**: 336–340.

Gersh, B.J., Stone, G.W., White, H.D., Holmes, DR., Jr. (2005). Pharmacological facilitation of primary percutaneous coronary intervention for acute myocardial infarction: is the slope of the curve the shape of the future? *JAMA*, **293**: 979–986.

Hausenloy, D.J., Yellon, D.M. (2006). Survival kinases in ischaemic preconditioning and postconditioning. *Cardiovasc Res*, **70**: 240–253.

He, K., Song, Y., Daviglus, M.L., *et al.,* (2004). Accumulated evidence on fish consumption and coronary heart disease mortality: a meta-analysis of cohort studies. *Circulation*, **109**: 2705–2711.

Lubbe, W.H., Podzuweit, T., Opie, L.H. (1992). Potential arrhythmogenic role of cyclic adenosine monophosphate (AMP) and cytosolic calcium overload: Implications for prophylactic effects of beta-blockers in myocardial infarction and proarrhythmic effects of phosphodiesterase inhibitors. *J Am Coll Cardiol*, **19**: 1622–1633.

Malmberg, K., Ryden, L., Efendic, S., *et al.,* (1995). Randomized trial of insulin-glucose infusion followed by subcutaneous insulin treatment in diabetic patients with acute myocardial infarction (DIGAMI Study): Effects on mortality at one year. *JACC*, **26**: 57–65.

Marchioli, R., Barzi, F., Bomba, E., *et al.,* (2002). Early protection against sudden death by n-3 polyunsaturated fatty acids after myocardial infarction: time-course analysis of the results of the Gruppo Italiano per lo Studio della Sopravvivenza nell'Infarto Miocardico (GISSI)-Prevenzione. *Circulation*, **105**: 1897–1903.

Mensah, K., Mocanu, M.M., Yellon, D.M. (2005). Failure to protect the myocardium against ischemia/reperfusion injury after chronic atorvastatin treatment is recaptured by acute atorvastatin treatment: a potential role for phosphatase and tensin homolog deleted on chromosome ten? *J Am Coll Cardiol*, **45**: 1287–1291.

Murphy, S.A., Gibson, C.M., Morrow, D.A., *et al.,* (2007). Efficacy and safety of the low-molecular weight heparin enoxaparin compared with unfractionated heparin across the acute coronary syndrome spectrum: a meta-analysis. *Eur Heart J*, **28**: 2077–2086.

Norris, R.M., Brown, M.A., Clarke, E.D., *et al.,* (1984). Prevention of ventricular fibrillation during acute myocardial infarction by intravenous propranolol. *Lancet*, **2**: 883–886.

Oliver, M.F., Kurien, V.A., Greenwood, T.W. (1968). Relation between serum free fatty acids and arrhythmias and death after myocardial infarction. *Lancet*, **1**: 710–715.

Opie, L., Pfeffer, M., (2008). Inhibitors of angiotensin-converting enzyme (ace), tensin-ii receptor, aldosterone, and renin. In: Opie LH, ed. *Drugs for the Heart*, 7th Edition, 2008: In press.

Opie, L.H. (1970). The glucose hypothesis: Relation to acute myocardial ischaemia. *J Mol Cell Cardiol*, **1**: 107–114.

Opie, L.H. (2007). Acute myocardial infarction and diabetes. *Lancet* 2007; **370**: 634–635.

Pratt, J.H. (2008). A not-so-modest proposal that a 'modest' increase in aldosterone causes hypertension and more. *Hypertension*, **51**: 39–40.

Roberts, R., Rogers, W.J., Mueller, H.S., *et al.*, (1991). For the TIMI Investigators. Immediate versus deferred β-blockade following thrombolytic therapy in patients with acute myocardial infarction. Results of the Thrombolysis in Myocardial Infarction (TIMI) II-B Study. *Circulation*, **83**: 422–437.

Staat, P., Rioufol, G., Piot, C., *et al.*, (2005). Postconditioning the human heart. *Circulation*, **112**: 2143–2148.

Van den Berghe, G., Wilmer, A., Hermans, G., *et al.*, (2006). Intensive insulin therapy in the medical ICU. *N Engl J Med*, **354**: 449–61.

Vetter, N.J., Adams, W., Strange, R.C., Oliver, M.F. (1974). Initial metabolic and hormonal response to acute myocardial infarction. *Lancet*, **1**: 284–248.

Yellon, D.M., Hausenloy, D.J. (2007). Myocardial reperfusion injury. *N Engl J Med*, **357**: 1121–1135.

Yellon, D.M., Opie, L.H. (2006). Postconditioning for protection of the infarcting heart. *Lancet*, **367**: 456–458.

Chapter 7

Cardioprotection During Cardiac Surgery

John Pepper

Key points

- Overall early mortality for cardiac surgery is low at 2–3% but in high risk patients it can be high as 10–15%
- The demography of cardiac surgical patients is changing to older and sicker patients
- Myocardial ischaemia-reperfusion injury and the systemic inflammatory response are closely related
- Several pharmacological agents that have been demonstrated to confer cardioprotection in the experimental setting have been applied to the clinical setting of cardiac surgery. However, the transfer of these findings from the bench to the bedside has been largely disappointing
- Potential cardioprotective strategies include pharmacological agents such as adenosine, and mechanical interventional strategies such as acute normovolaemic haemodilution and remote ischaemic preconditioning.

7.1 Introduction

The objective of every cardiac operation should be a technically perfect result without producing myocardial damage. The pre-requisites for optimal cardioprotection are uniform and adequate distribution of a cardioprotective agent, excellent visualisation of the operative field, a simple technique that does not distract the surgeon, and optimal protection of the brain and kidneys. The consequences of inadequate cardioprotection range from low cardiac output states leading to multi-organ failure, increased mortality and prolonged ICU and hospital stay; to subtle degrees of damage causing delayed myocardial fibrosis. In patients with pre-operative impaired left ventricular function the margins of functional reserve are narrow and methods of cardioprotection have therefore to be focused. Recently much debate has occurred about the relative merits of on-pump and off-pump surgery and whether the avoidance of a period of extracorporeal perfusion is beneficial to the myocardium. This debate remains unresolved, but in expert hands equivalent results can be obtained by both techniques.

7.2 **Cardioplegia and cross-clamp fibrillation**

The basic principles of cardioprotection in the cardiac surgical setting are: rapid cardiac arrest, hypothermia and the avoidance of myocardial oedema. Most surgeons use blood cardioplegia to provide additional substrate, oxygen, improved buffering and anti-oxidants; and they employ a combination of antegrade and retrograde delivery systems. Despite numerous reports, there have been no definitive prospective studies that narrow the methods enough to allow universal adoption of one particular technique. Results for low risk operations are satisfactory using cold blood cardioplegia delivered by a combination of antegrade and retrograde routes. Cross-clamp fibrillation represents another technique for myocardial preservation that is used in increasingly fewer patients.

As a result of surgically induced myocardial ischaemia by aortic cross-clamping, there is a cessation or attenuation of coronary blood flow such that oxygen delivery to the myocardium is insufficient to meet basal myocardial requirements to preserve cell membrane viability. Recovery involves a resumption of normal oxidative metabolism and the restoration of myocardial energy reserves. In addition there is a reversal of ischaemia-induced cell swelling and loss of membrane ion gradients and the adenine nucleotide pool. Finally, there is the need to repair damaged cell organelles such as the mitochondria and the sarcoplasmic reticulum. Despite meticulous adherence to known principles of cardioprotection, such patients may require inotropic support and mechanical assistance in the form of intra-aortic balloon pumps or short-term ventricular assist devices.

Perhaps the most challenging group of patients are those with concentric left ventricular hypertrophy due to aortic stenosis combined with three vessel coronary artery disease. Attention to detail is required to prevent significant myocardial injury in this high-risk patient group. Another difficult group of patients are re-operations particularly when the prior operation has occurred in an era when cardioprotection was less developed. Such patients may have old subendocardial infarcts which can be identified pre-operatively by gadolinium enhanced magnetic resonance imaging (Figure 7.1). Finally, those patients who have impaired left ventricular function and ischaemic mitral regurgitation represent a high risk group with a EURO score often over 20.

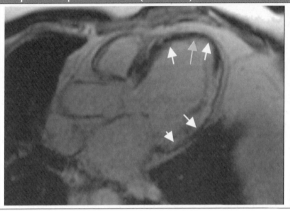

Figure 7.1 Poor LV, Aortic stenosis, Previous MI (subendocardial mainly –white arrows – but transmural at apex with apical thrombus (red arrow)

7.3 Minimizing cardiopulmonary bypass

The standard prime volume for the cardiopulmonary bypass circuit is 1500 mls of crystalloid solution. Use of low-prime circuits with reduced volumes of 500 ml may have a positive effect on the inflammatory response and are the subject of intense investigation. The standard heart-lung bypass machine can be a major trigger of inflammatory reactions potentially inducing organ failure including myocardial damage (Asimakopoulos, 1999). New ideas of reduction of the artificial surface area, reducing the blood-air interface and optimisation of surface coating may lead to real improvements in myocardial protection. In a randomized study of 60 patients undergoing CABG surgery, Skrabal et al., (2007) compared a novel minimal extracorporeal circuit (MECC) with conventional cardiopulmonary bypass on myocardial injury. The MECC group demonstrated significantly lower levels of Troponin T (ng/ml) at 6, 12 and 24 hours (0.07 ± 0.01 vs. 0.16 ± 0.04 $p<0.005$; 0.12 ± 0.03 vs. 0.28 ± 0.08 $p<0.008$; 0.21 ± 0.05 vs. 0.35 ± 0.09 $p< 0.03$, respectively). In a larger prospective, non-randomized study of 136 consecutive patients undergoing CABG surgery, 54 patients (39.7%) were operated with a mini-prime extracorporeal circuit (mini-ECC) (Immer et al., 2005). Post-operative CK-MB and Troponin I were significantly lower in the mini-ECC group ($p <0.05$) and the requirement for inotropic support and incidence of post-operative atrial fibrillation were significantly lower. In most of these mini-prime extracorporeal circuits the heart is not completely unloaded and there is minimal residual perfusion of the arrested heart which could be one explanation for improved protection because it eliminates, almost completely, the presence of air in the coronary system.

7.4 Off-pump surgery

The avoidance of cardiopulmonary bypass by the use of off-pump techniques has not resulted in a clear benefit in terms of reduced mortality or reduced incidence of peri-operative myocardial infarction. However, most observers have reported a significant reduction in Troponin T release. Although there is enormous enthusiasm for off-pump CABG surgery in some quarters, the overall uptake has been about 20% across the board. Using high fidelity LV pressure recordings combined with 2-D echo recordings from peri-operative transoesophageal echocardiography, we have shown a remarkable tolerance of the myocardium to occlusion of the left anterior descending artery for periods of up to 15 minutes (Figure 7.2) (Koh et al., 1999). In the presence of collaterals from a dominant right coronary artery, there is very little change in myocardial contractility as revealed by analysis of anterior wall-thickening. In the absence of collaterals, normal wall thickening is restored within 10 minutes. This type of surgery requires a different surgical approach. Careful, individualised choice of graft sequence and maintenance of stable systemic haemodynamics are fundamental (Puskas et al., 2001). It is important to graft the collateralised vessel or vessels first and to reperfuse these by performing proximal anastomoses or releasing clamps on the internal mammary artery pedicles. The collateralizing vessel can then be safely grafted. In this way, vital coronary flow provided by collateralising vessels is not interrupted. In general, peri-operative myocardial ischaemia is less pronounced in off-pump coronary artery bypass (OPCAB) compared to on-pump surgery. However, the degree of cardiac Troponin I (cTnI) and creatine kinase-MB (CK-MB) released during OPCAB, which should be considered clinically important, is currently unknown. Paperalla et al., (2007) examined this problem in a prospective series of 261 patients undergoing OPCAB surgery. The degree of postoperative cTnI and CK-MB elevation did not predict in-hospital mortality and the incidence of low cardiac output. However, the survival rate over 3 years was significantly worse in patients with the highest postoperative peak release of cTnI and CK-MB. Adjusted hazard ratios for 3-year mortality were HR 2.7 (CI 1–7.6), p = 0.05 for cTnI >7.1 ng/dl and HR 3.1 (CI 1–9.1), p = 0.04 for CK-MB >36.3 ng/ml. They concluded that peri-operative myocardial damage should not be considered an innocuous even In the myocardium.

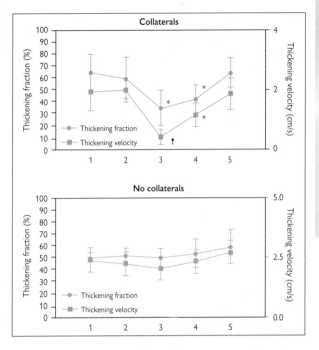

Figure 7.2 Results of occluding the LAD on anterior wall-thickening during beating heart surgery. Note the rapid resolution of this injury. 1 = baseline, 2 = stabilization, 3 = occlusion, 4 = 2 mins post snare release, 5 =10 mins post snare release.

7.5 **Acute Normovolaemic Haemodilution**

This technique allows blood viscosity to be lowered, thereby facilitating blood flow through diseased coronary vessels, collaterals and ischaemic myocardium. A small clinical study of 84 patients reported that acute normovolaemic haemodilution (ANV to achieve a haematocrit of 28%) was able to reduce myocardial injury as measured by serum troponin I in both patients undergoing CABG surgery (Licker et al., 2005) and in patients with LV hypertrophy undergoing aortic valve replacement (Licker et al., 2007).

7.6 **Endogenous Forms of Cardioprotection**

7.6.1 **Ischaemic Preconditioning**

Ischaemic preconditioning (IPC) refers to a powerful endogenous form of cardioprotection, which is elicited by subjecting the myocardium to one or more transient non-lethal episodes of myocardial ischaemia and reperfusion (Murry *et al.,* 1986). Jenkins *et al.,* (1997) were the first to demonstrate its efficacy during CABG surgery, using invasive cross-clamping of the aorta as the preconditioning stimulus. The protection offered by classical preconditioning lasts 2 to 3 hours but the second window of preconditioning (Yellon & Downey 2003) whose protection lasts for 24 to 96 hours may offer a greater clinical benefit. In practice, ischaemic preconditioning induced by repetitive cross clamping of the ascending aorta is very unattractive especially in an ageing patient population with advanced atherosclerosis because of the risk of thromboembolism. In the setting of off-pump surgery in the early days, ischaemic preconditioning seemed appropriate and acceptable for single vessel bypass via small thoracotomy (MIDCAB) but as the number of bypass grafts performed during OPCAB increased, enthusiasm of surgeons to perform repeated episodes of ischaemic preconditioning to each coronary artery waned. IPC can also be mimicked in the experimental setting by vigorous beta-adrenergic stimulation, cycles of calcium depletion and repletion, rapid cardiac pacing, hypoxia or stretch of cardiomyocytes and inhalational anaesthetics. Therefore, during the journey that a patient follows from ward to anaesthetic room to the operating theatre there are probably multiple stimuli contributing to a potential preconditioning effect (see later section for pharmacological agents which have been examined as preconditioning mimetics in the setting of cardiac surgery).

7.6.2 **Remote Ischaemic Preconditioning**

Compared to IPC which necessitates an intervention applied directly to the heart, remote ischaemic preconditioning (RIPC) provides a more amenable and less-invasive cardioprotective strategy. This describes the intriguing phenomenon in which the application of one or more brief episodes of ischaemia and reperfusion in one tissue or organ, such as the small intestine, kidney, liver or limb, protects a distant tissue or organ such as the heart from a more sustained episode of ischaemia (Przyklenk *et al.,* 1993). Hausenloy *et al.,* (2007) recently carried out a clinical study in adults undergoing elective CABG surgery investigating the effects of RIPC using transient ischaemia of the arm. Patients were randomized to receive either RIPC, comprising three-5 min cycles of cuff inflation and deflation (N = 27), or control (N = 30; cuff positioned but not inflated). Serum troponin T was sequentially measured after surgery; the total area under the curve was reduced by 43% in the intervention group. This is clearly a powerful endogenous cardioprotective system which should be harnessed to improve myocardial protection. Larger clinical studies are required to determine whether there are any beneficial effects on clinical outcomes following surgery.

7.7 Pharmacological cardioprotection

In an attempt to improve clinical outcomes in patients undergoing cardiac surgery, several pharmacological treatment strategies, which have been demonstrated in experimental studies to confer cardio-protection, have been examined in the clinical setting. Clearly, any such treatment strategy would have to prove itself capable of limiting myocardial injury over and above that provided by current cardio-protective strategies such as cardioplegia.

Inhalational anaesthetics have been extensively investigated in the clinical setting of cardiac surgery as a potential cardioprotective agent. These agents, which include isofurane and desflurane, have been reported to mimic the cardioprotection elicited by IPC, recruiting similar signal transduction pathways. Although several clinical studies have demonstrated a reduction in myocardial injury as measured by the release of cardiac enzymes and improved morbidity, a recent meta-analysis failed to find any beneficial effects on AMI and mortality in CABG patients (Symons & Myles, 2006).

During myocardial ischaemia the acidic conditions generated by lactate accumulation promote intracellular calcium loading, a process which can be attenuated by pharmacologically inhibiting the sarcolemmal Na^+-H^+ exchanger (NHE) in experimental studies. Recent efforts to reduce the impact of myocardial ischaemia-reperfusion injury during cardiac surgery have concentrated on the inhibition of the NHE using the pharmacological agent, cariporide (Boyce et al., 2003). A large randomized clinical trial (GUARDIAN) suggested benefits of NHE inhibition in high-risk cardiac surgery. However, a subsequent randomized trial of cardiac surgery (EXPEDITION) had to be terminated early because of a significantly increased incidence of cere-brovascular events from 2.7% in the placebo group to 4.8% in the cariporide-treated group (p <0.001) (Mentzer et al., 2003). Thus, although experimental studies were very encouraging, clinical trials have been disappointing.

In contrast, clinical trials of the use of adenosine and it agonist in CABG surgery (Menzter et al., 1999) have been more encouraging. Experimental studies have clearly demonstrated that adenosine, which is generated during myocardial ischaemia, confers powerful cardioprotection through its action as a preconditioning mimetic in addition to its anti-inflammatory effects. In addition to it being added to cardioplegic solution, the administration of adenosine as an intra-venous infusion prior to cardiac surgery was demonstrated to reduce the need for high-dose inotropes and decrease the development of peri-operative MI (Menzter et al., 1999). A large multi-centred 2698 patient trial investigating the pre-treatment with an intravenous infu-sion of acadesine, an agent which augments levels of adenosine in ischaemic tissue, failed to report any beneficial effects of the primary endpoint of cardiac death, AMI, or stroke at 4 days in CABG patients (Mangano *et al.*, 2006). However, in a small subgroup of patients that experienced a peri-operative AMI (N = 100), those that had received acadesine sustained markedly reduced mortality rates at 2 years (27.8% with acadesine versus 6.5% with placebo; p = 0.006).

It is a common observation in high-risk surgical patients that a severe inflammatory response (SIRS) develops in the early post-operative period which leads to a prolonged stay in the intensive care unit and is accompanied by the need for renal and prolong respiratory support. There have been several attempts to ameliorate the SIRS effect including the inhibition of the complement cascade. The PRIMO-CABG study examined the effect of the C5 complement inhibitor, pexelizumab, in a multi-centred phase III randomized controlled clinical trial comprising 3,099 patients undergoing cardiac surgery (Verrier *et al.*, 2004). There was no difference in the primary composite end point comprising the incidence of death or AMI within 30 days of surgery (9.8% with pexelizumab versus 11.8% with placebo (relative risk, 0.82; 95% confidence interval, 0.66–1.02; P = .07) in patients undergoing CABG surgery only. However, in the intent-to-treat analyses, which included patients undergoing valve surgery in addition to CABG surgery, there was a significant reduction in this composite end-point (11.5% with pexelizumab versus 14.0% receiving placebo; relative risk, 0.82; 95% confidence interval, 0.68–0.99; P = .03). The trial had not been powered to detect a reduction in mortality alone. A further prospective randomized trial demonstrating a reduction will be required before this treatment can be routinely adopted by cardiac surgeons.

7.8 **Conclusions**

Cardioprotection remains an important issue in cardiac surgery especially in view of the changing demography with both older and sicker patients being operated on. For brief, straightforward procedures with well-preserved left ventricular function, current techniques are adequate. Complex procedures with ischaemic times over two hours require additional measures. Careful, targeted, randomized clinical trials investigating new cardioprotective strategies are required if our patients are to benefit from translational research.

Key references

Asimakopoulos, G. (1999). Mechanisms of the systemic inflammatory response. *Perfusion*, **14**: 269–277.

Boyce, S.W., Bartels, C., Bolli, R., et al., (2003). GUARD during ischemia against necrosis (GUARDIAN) Study Investigators. Impact of sodium-hydrogen exchange inhibition on death or myocardial infarction in high risk CABG patients: results of the CABG surgery cohort of the GUARDIAN study. *J Thorac Cardiovasc Surg*, **126**: 420–427.

Hausenloy, D.J., Mwamure, P.K., Venugopal, V., et al., (2007). Effect of remote ischaemic preconditioning in patients undergoing coronary artery bypass graft surgery: a randomized trial. *Lancet*, **370**: 575–579.

Immer, F.F., Pirovino, C., Gygax, E., et al., (2005). Minimal versus conventional cardiopulmonary bypass: assessment of intraoperative myocardial damage in coronary bypass surgery. *Eur J Cardiothorac Surg*, **28**: 701–704.

Jenkins, D.P., Pugsley, W.B., Alkhulaifi, A.M., et al., (1997). Ischaemic preconditioning reduces troponin T release in patients undergoing coronary artery bypass surgery. *Heart*, **77**: 314–318.

Koh, T.W., Carr-White. G.S., DeSouza, A.C., et al., (1999). Effect of coronary occlusion on left ventricular function with and without collateral supply during beating heart coronary artery surgery. *Heart*, **81**: 285–291.

Licker, M., Ellenberger, C., Sierra, J., et al., (2005). Cardioprotective effects of acute normovolemic hemodilution in patients undergoing coronary artery bypass surgery. *Chest*, **128**: 838–847.

Licker, M., Sierra, J., Kalangos, A., et al., (2007). Cardioprotective effects of acute normovolemic hemodilution in patients with severe aortic stenosis undergoing valve replacement. *Transfusion*, **47**: 341–350.

Mangano, D.T., Miao, Y., Tudor, I.C., et al., (2006). Post-reperfusion myocardial infarction: long-term survival improvement using adenosine regulation with acadesine. *J Am Coll Cardiol*, **48**: 206–214.

Mentzer, R.M., Birjiniuk, V., Khuri, S., et al., (1999). Adenosine myocardial protection: preliminary results of a phase II clinical trial. *Ann Thorac Surg*, **229**: 643–649.

Mentzer, R.M., the EXPEDITION Study Investigators. (2003). Effects of Na^+/H^+ exchange inhibition by cariporide on death and non-fatal myocardial infarction in patients undergoing coronary artery bypass graft surgery: The EXPEDITION Study. *Circulation*, **108**: 3M.

Murry, C.E., Jennings, R.B., Reimer, K.A. (1986). Preconditioning with ischaemia: a delay of lethal cell injury in ischemic myocardium. *Circulation*, **74**: 1124–1136.

Paperalla, D., Cappabianca, G., Malvindi, P., et al., (2007). Myocardial injury after off-pump coronary artery bypass grafting operation. *Eur J Cardiothorac Surg*, **32**: 481–487.

Przyklenk, K., Bauer, B., Ovize, M., et al., (1993). Regional ischemic 'preconditioning' protects remote virgin myocardium from subsequent sustained coronary occlusion. *Circulation*, **87**: 893–899.

Puskas, J.D., Vinten-Johansen, J., Muraki, S., Guyton, R.A. (2001). Myocardial protection for off-pump coronary bypass surgery. *Semin Thorac Cardiovasc Surg*, **13**: 82–88.

Skrabal, C.A., Steinhoff, G., Liebold, A. (2007). Minimising cardiopulmonary bypass attenuates myocardial damage after cardiac surgery. *ASAIO J*, **53**: 32–35.

Symons, J.A., Myles, P.S. (2006). Myocardial protection with volatile anaesthetic agents during coronary artery bypass surgery: a meta-analysis. *Br J Anaesth*, **97**: 127–136.

Verrier, E.D., Shernan, S.K., Taylor, K.M., *et al.,* (2004). Terminal complement blockade with pexelizumab during coronary artery bypass graft surgery requiring cardiopulmonary bypass: randomized trial. *JAMA*, **291**: 2319–2327.

Yellon, D.M., Downey J.M. (2003). Preconditioning the myocardium: from cellular physiology to clinical cardiology. *Physiol Rev*, **83**: 1113–1151.

Chapter 8

Endogenous Mechanisms of Cardioprotection

James Downey & Michael Cohen

Key points

- Ischaemic preconditioning is the most powerful endogenous mechanism for limiting myocardial infarct size in the experimental setting. Its clinical application is limited to scenarios in which the index episode of ischaemia and reperfusion can be anticipated such as in the setting of cardiac surgery
- Ischaemic postconditioning represents an endogenous cardioprotective strategy which is applied at the onset of myocardial reperfusion, thereby allowing its use as an adjunct to reperfusion in patients presenting with an acute myocardial infarction
- Both ischaemic preconditioning and postconditioning recruit a common signal transduction pathway at the time of myocardial reperfusion, which can be targeted by pharmacological agents administered as adjuncts to reperfusion.

8.1 Endogenous cardioprotection

The heart possesses the ability to protect itself against the detrimental effects of ischaemia-reperfusion injury. This endogenous adaptive state requires a preconditioning stimulus comprising one or more short-lived episodes of myocardial ischaemia and reperfusion – and was termed Ischaemic Preconditioning (IPC) in 1986 in a seminal study by Murry et al., (1986). It transpires that the resistance against ischaemia-reperfusion can also be elicited by applying the preconditioning ischaemia to an organ or tissue remote from the heart- a phenomenon termed Remote Ischaemic Preconditioning (RIPC), (Pryzklenk et al., 1993). However, it is important to appreciate that an intervention which needs to be applied prior to the injurious ischaemic event, as in the case of IPC, is limited in application to situations in which the ischaemia can be reliably anticipated such as in cardiac surgery.

The introduction of ischaemic postconditioning surmounts this obstacle to translation by providing an intervention which can be applied at the onset of reperfusion and therefore can be applied to patients presenting with an AMI (Zhao et al., 2003). In this scenario, the process of myocardial reperfusion is interrupted with several short-lived episodes of myocardial ischaemia- inducing a stuttered form of myocardial reperfusion. Finally, the cardioprotection elicited by RIPC can also be applied after the onset of myocardial ischaemia and immediately prior to reperfusion, making remote ischaemic post-conditioning (RIPost), as it has been termed (Kerendi et al., 2005), a potential cardioprotective intervention for AMI patients.

8.2 Ischaemic preconditioning

Although reperfusion therapy is effective at limiting infarct size and reducing the incidence of heart failure in patients experiencing acute myocardial infarction, it seldom can be instituted soon enough to prevent significant necrosis. Thus there has been a quest to find some agent that would make the ischaemic heart resistant to infarction so that less tissue would be lost for any duration of ischaemia. As mentioned above β-blockers and free radical scavengers were inconsistent in their ability to protect and even the positive studies reported only a modest degree of salvage. Then in 1986, Murry et al., (Murry, Jennings & Reimer, 1986) reported that preconditioning a dog heart with 4 cycles of 5 min of coronary artery occlusion followed by 5 min of reperfusion prior to a 40-min coronary occlusion resulted in a much smaller infarct than seen with the occlusion alone (Figure 8.1).

The short periods of ischaemia caused the heart to adapt itself to become very resistant to myocardial infarction. Also the magnitude of the protection was striking as infarcts in the preconditioned hearts were only about 1/4 of those seen in untreated hearts despite the fact that the preconditioned hearts had endured an additional 20 min of ischaemia. All who have tried to duplicate ischaemic preconditioning (IPC) have seen essentially the same result. Furthermore it seemed to work equally well in all species tested. This was the first demonstration that cardioprotection was actually possible and so the quest began to try to find a way to translate this protection to the cardiac patient.

8.2.1 Mechanism of IPC – the trigger phase

Now that two decades have passed since its discovery we have a fairly good understanding of how IPC works. Figure 8.2 shows a flow chart of the signal transduction steps that have been identified to date in IPC. During the preconditioning ischaemia several autacoids are

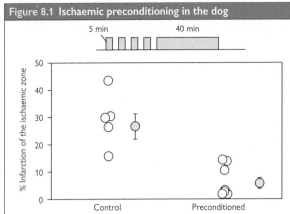

Figure 8.1 Ischaemic preconditioning in the dog

5 min   40 min

% Infarction of the ischaemic zone

Control   Preconditioned

Open-chested dogs underwent 40 min coronary artery occlusion followed by reperfusion. Infarct size is expressed as a % of the ischaemic risk zone on the vertical axis. Open symbols show individual experiments and solid symbols group mean ± SEM. Note that 4 cycles of 5 min occlusion + 5 min reperfusion (ischaemic preconditioning) made the heart very resistant to infarction as compared to control hearts. From Murry et al., (Murry, Jennings, & Reimer, 1986).

released by the myocytes including adenosine, bradykinin and an endogenous opioid endorphin. These populate G_i-coupled receptors on the cardiomyocyte which, through varying pathways, converge on a signalling molecule called protein kinase C (PKC). Interestingly, bradykinin and opioid receptors couple to PKC through the opening of potassium channels in the inner membrane of the heart's mitochondria causing them to produce oxygen-based free radicals. These radicals act as second messengers to activate PKC. The ischaemic cycle is required to produce the autacoids that open the channels while the reperfusion cycle is then thought to supply the oxygen needed to make the signalling radicals. Giving any of the autacoids to the heart prior to ischaemia mimics the protection of IPC – so-called 'pharmacological preconditioning'. We call this the "trigger phase" since transient exposure to an autacoid puts the heart into the protected state which will persist for about an hour or two even after the autacoid is washed out.

8.2.2 Mechanism of IPC – mPTP inhibition

There is now overwhelming evidence that the actual protective event in IPC is the inhibition of mitochondrial permeability transition pore (mPTP) opening following the lethal ischaemic insult (Hausenloy et al., 2002). Only recently have investigators tried to unravel events in the mediator-effector pathway. The overall scheme can be summarized as follows: Redox signalling following reperfusion keeps PKC active.

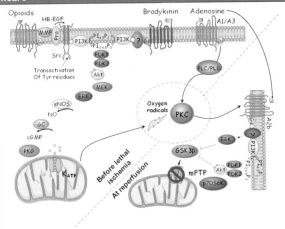

Figure 8.2 Signal transduction pathways in the preconditioned heart

Opioid and bradykinin receptors trigger protection by opening a potassium channel in the mitochondria resulting in activation of PKC through a burst of oxygen radicals. Adenosine A_1 receptors directly activate PKC through phospholipases. At reperfusion the A_{2B} receptors are thought to be sensitized by PKC so that endogenous adenosine can populate them. The A_{2B} receptors inhibit mPTP formation through their coupling to Akt, ERK and GSK3B. From Tissier et al. (Tissier, Cohen & Downey, 2007).

PKC in turn is thought to sensitise the heart's adenosine A_{2B} receptors to respond to endogenously produced adenosine. The reperfused heart has an elevated adenosine level but it is not high enough to populate the very low-affinity adenosine A_{2B} receptors unless they have been sensitized by PKC. The heart's A_{2B} receptors couple to two survival kinase systems: extracellular signal-related kinase (ERK) and the phosphatidylinositol 3-kinase (PI3-K)/Akt pathway- termed the Reperfusion Injury Salvage Kinase (RISK) pathway (Hausenloy & Yellon, 2004). These kinases somehow exert an inhibitory influence on mPTP formation, possibly through another downstream kinase glycogen synthase kinase-3β (GSK-3β).

Animal studies reveal that following a period of myocardial ischaemia, forces within the injured cell try to open the mPTP during the first hour of reperfusion (Solenkova et al., 2006). Signals from the protective pathways must be in place from the first seconds of reperfusion and must be continuously present until the heart has repaired the ischaemic injury, which takes about 60 minutes in a rabbit's heart. Any interruption of the protective pathways during the convalescent hour results in mPTP opening and necrosis.

8.2.3 Mechanism of IPC–protection at time of reperfusion

It was originally thought that preconditioning could only be instituted prior to ischaemia. The requirement for pre-treatment limited its use to iatrogenic ischaemia such as that which occurs in cardiac surgery and cardiac transplantation. However, for those settings powerful cardioplegic agents are already available. As a result IPC had little clinical impact. With the discovery that IPC exerts its actual protection during reperfusion (Hausenloy et al., 2005), it became apparent that IPC's protection theoretically could still be conferred right up to the time of reperfusion. A growing list of pharmacological agents has now been identified that can effectively put the heart into a preconditioned state when given just prior to reperfusion. Among those are transforming growth factor-β, erythropoietin, natriuretic peptides, bradykinin, opioid-δ agonists, A_{2B}-selective adenosine agonists, PKG activators, and even 'statins'. A number of these have been examined in the clinical setting of an AMI (see Chapter 11).

8.3 Second window of protection

When a heart is preconditioned the initial protection is short-lived and wanes within an hour or two of the preconditioning stimulus. However, the protection is seen to return within 24 h of the insult and lasts for up to 4 days (Baxter, Goma & Yellon, 1997). This second window of preconditioning (SWOP), which was first described by Marber et al., (1993), is less potent than seen in the first window and is thought to be the result of expression of protective genes including inducible nitric oxide synthase (iNOS) and cyclooxygenase 2 (COX2) (Bolli, Dawn & Xuan, 2003). The attractiveness of the second window is that a single treatment provides days of protection, and that might be useful for protecting high-risk patients. Dana et al., (Dana et al., 1998) found that rabbits could be protected indefinitely if they were preconditioned with a bolus of an adenosine A_1 agonist at 2-day intervals. Although SWOP is attractive, the logistics of designing a clinical trial that would include enough events to achieve statistical power proved to be overwhelming. As a result second window interventions have never been tested in man.

8.4 Remote ischaemic preconditioning

There have been several reports that preconditioning one region of the heart offers protection to another region (Pryzklenk et al., 1993). Furthermore preconditioning another organ can even protect the heart. The inference is that some unknown humoral or neural signal is activated by the preconditioned organ which then targets the heart. This may have practical clinical value as preconditioning the arm with a blood pressure cuff was reported to protect the hearts of patients undergoing coronary artery bypass grafting (Hausenloy et al., 2007). Importantly, remote preconditioning will still protect when instituted after myocardial ischaemia suggesting that it may be applied to the clinical setting of an AMI.

8.5 Ischaemic postconditioning

In 2003, Vinten-Johansen's group described experiments with post-conditioning (Zhao et al., 2003). They tested whether reperfusion/ occlusion cycles applied at reperfusion might be as protective as those prior to ischaemia. Surprisingly they were found to be just as protective (see Figure 8.3). The duration of the cycles had to be decreased from 5 min to 30 sec in the canine heart and even to 10 sec in the isolated rodent heart. At first it was thought that the mechanism was unrelated to that for IPC, but then it was noted that inhibitors of ERK or PI3-K could abort the protection just as was seen in IPC (Yang et al., 2004). It now appears that the staccato reperfusion adds enough oxygen to promote redox signalling while at the same time keeping perfusion low enough to keep the tissue acidotic (Cohen, Yang & Downey, 2007). The mPTP does not form until reperfusion because the low pH during ischaemia inhibits its formation. The intermittent ischaemia keeps the mPTP closed due to the acidosis and thus provides enough time for redox signalling to precondition the heart and put the signals in place to inhibit mPTP even after the reperfusion/ischaemia cycles are stopped and pH normalises. The requirements for postconditioning in a rabbit heart are that the first occlusion be instituted no longer than 30 sec after opening the artery and that the cycles be continued for at least 2 min. The reperfusion cycles should not be so long as to allow pH to normalize. Shorter cycles are better, but 30 sec occlusions and reperfusions work well for in situ rabbits.

The advantage of postconditioning is that it lends itself well to patients that are reperfused with primary angioplasty. In a recent clinical trial Staat et al., (Staat et al., 2005) recanalized the occluded artery by deploying a stent in the region of the thrombus. Half of the 30 patients were then subjected to 4 cycles of 1 min reperfusion followed by 1 min balloon inflation to reocclude the artery, while the other half received no additional balloon inflations. Among other parameters postconditioning produced a 36% reduction of infarct size as determined by enzyme release (see chapter 11 for further details).

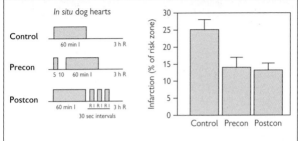

Figure 8.3 Ischaemic preconditioning (precon) compared to postconditioning (postcon) in the dog heart

The experimental protocol appears on the left. Shaded areas represent periods of coronary branch occlusion. Note that three 30-sec cycles of postconditioning was equipotent with preconditioning at reducing infarct size. From Zhao et al., (Zhao, Corvera, Halkos, Kerendi, Wang, Guyton & Vinten-Johansen 2003). Used with permission.

8.6 **Conclusions**

'Conditioning' the heart adapts it to withstand ischaemia-reperfusion injury. This endogenous form of cardioprotection can be elicited by subjecting the heart (ischaemic preconditioning) or an organ or tissue remote from the heart (remote ischaemic preconditioning), to one or more transient episodes of myocardial ischaemia and reperfusion. However, its clinical utility is limited to clinical settings in which the index ischaemic episode can be anticipated such as in cardiac bypass surgery.

A more clinically relevant intervention for patients presenting with an acute myocardial infarction, is ischaemic postconditioning, in which normal myocardial reperfusion is interrupted by several short-lived episodes of myocardial ischaemia. The application of brief ischaemia and reperfusion to an organ or tissue remote from the heart after the onset of a myocardial infarction but prior to myocardial reperfusion has been termed remote ischaemic postconditioning. Of particular note, is that these mechanical strategies of cardioprotection can be reproduced by pharmacological agents directed to the underlying signal transduction pathways, thereby obviating the need for an invasive cardioprotective strategy.

Key References

Baxter, G.F., Goma, F.M., Yellon, D. M. (1997). Characterisation of the infarct-limiting effect of delayed preconditioning: timecourse and dose-dependency studies in rabbit myocardium. *Basic Res. Cardiol*, **92**: 159–167.

Bolli, R., Dawn, B., Xuan, Y.T. (2003). Role of the JAK-STAT pathway in protection against myocardial ischemia/reperfusion injury. *Trends Cardiovasc Med*, **13**: 72–79.

Cohen, M.V., Yang, X.M., Downey, J.M. (2007). The pH hypothesis of postconditioning: staccato reperfusion reintroduces oxygen and perpetuates myocardial acidosis. *Circulation*, **115**: 1895–1903.

Dana, A., Baxter, G.F., Walker, J.M., Yellon, D.M. (1998). Prolonging the delayed phase of myocardial protection: repetitive adenosine A_1 receptor activation maintains rabbit myocardium in a preconditioned state. *J Am Coll Cardiol*, **31**: 1142–1149.

Hausenloy, D.J., Maddock, H.L., Baxter, G.F., Yellon, D.M. (2002). Inhibiting mitochondrial permeability transition pore opening: a new paradigm for myocardial preconditioning? *Cardiovasc Res*, **55**: 534–543.

Hausenloy, D.J., Yellon, D.M. (2004). New directions for protecting the heart against ischaemia-reperfusion injury: targeting the Reperfusion Injury Salvage Kinase (RISK)-pathway. *Cardiovasc Res*, **61**: 448–460.

Hausenloy, D.J., Tsang, A., Mocanu, M., Yellon, D.M. (2005). Ischemic preconditioning protects by activating pro-survival kinases at reperfusion. *Am J Physiol Heart Circ Physiol*, **288**: H971–H976.

Hausenloy, D.J., Mwamure, P.K., Harris, J., *et al.*, (2007). Effect of remote ischaemic preconditioning on myocardial injury in patients undergoing coronary artery bypass graft surgery: a randomized controlled trial. *Lancet*, **370**: 575–579.

Hearse, D.J., Yellon, D.M., Downey, J.M. (1986). Can beta blockers limit myocardial infarct size? *Eur. Heart J*, **7**: 925–930.

Kerendi, F., Kin, H., Halkos, M.E., *et al.*, (2005). Remote postconditioning. Brief renal ischemia and reperfusion applied before coronary artery reperfusion reduces myocardial infarct size via endogenous activation of adenosine receptors. *Basic Res Cardiol*, **100**: 404–412.

Marber, M.S., Latchman, D.S., Walker, J.M., Yellon, D.M. (1993). Cardiac stress protein elevation 24 hours after brief ischemia or heat stress is associated with resistance to myocardial infarction. *Circulation*, **88**: 1264–1272.

Mehta, S.R., Yusuf, S., Diaz, R., *et al.*, (2005). Effect of glucose-insulin-potassium infusion on mortality in patients with acute ST-segment elevation myocardial infarction: the CREATE-ECLA randomized controlled trial. *JAMA*, **293**: 437–446.

Murry, C.E., Jennings, R.B., Reimer, K.A. (1986). Preconditioning with ischemia: a delay of lethal cell injury in ischemic myocardium. *Circulation*, **74**: 1124–1136.

Przyklenk, K., Bauer, B., Ovize, M., *et al.*, (1993). Regional ischemic 'preconditioning' protects remote virgin myocardium from subsequent sustained coronary occlusion. *Circulation*, **87**: 893–899.

Solenkova, N.V., Solodushko, V., Cohen, M.V., Downey, J.M. (2006). Endogenous adenosine protects preconditioned heart during early minutes of reperfusion by activating Akt. *Am J Physiol*, **290**: H441–H449.

Staat, P., Rioufol, G., Piot, C., *et al.*, (2005). Postconditioning the human heart. *Circulation*, **112**: 2143–2148.

Tissier, R., Cohen, M.V., Downey, J.M. (2007). Protecting the acutely ischemic myocardium beyond reperfusion therapies: are we any closer to realizing the dream of infarct size elimination? *Arch Mal Coeur Vaiss,* **100**(9): 794–802. Elsevier Masson.

Yang, X.M., Proctor, J.B., Cui, *et al.*, (2004). Multiple, brief coronary occlusions during early reperfusion protect rabbit hearts by targeting cell signaling pathways. *J Am Coll Cardiol*, **44**: 1103–1110.

Yang, Z., Day, Y.J., Toufektsian, M.C., *et al.*, (2005). Infarct-sparing effect of A2A-adenosine receptor activation is due primarily to its action on lymphocytes. *Circulation*, **111**: 2190–2197.

Zhao, Z.Q., Corvera, J.S., Halkos, *et al.*, (2003). Inhibition of myocardial injury by ischemic postconditioning during reperfusion: comparison with ischemic preconditioning. *Am J Physiol*, **285**: H579–H588.

Chapter 9

Adjunctive Reperfusion Therapy Post-AMI

Thorsten Reffelmann & Robert Kloner

Key points

- Reperfusion of the occluded coronary artery in an ST-segment-elevation myocardial infarction is the most effective approach for reducing infarct size, preserving left ventricular ejection fraction, lowering the incidence and severity of congestive heart failure and improving prognosis

- Hence, several pharmacologic agents intended to improve target vessel patency as an adjunct to thrombolysis or primary percutaneous coronary intervention have been shown to be beneficial in patients with reperfusion therapy for acute myocardial infarction, namely antiplatelet and anticoagulation agents

- Animal investigations have suggested that coronary reperfusion may also result in undesirable cardiac alterations, termed 'reperfusion injury', such as reversible contractile dysfunction ('stunning'), microvascular obstruction ('no-reflow'), and in several studies the progression of myocardial necrosis ('lethal reperfusion injury')

- Clinical investigations of various pharmacologic interventions as an adjunctive therapy to reperfusion to reduce final infarct size, the amount of contractile dysfunction and to improve prognosis have been mostly inconsistent; only a few interventions, e.g. adenosine and atrial natriuretic peptide seem to show promise at least in certain subgroups.

9.1 Early reperfusion – the prerequisite for infarct size reduction

Early coronary reperfusion in acute ST-segment elevation myocardial infarction has consistently been shown to reduce infarct size and improve prognosis (Figure 9.1). Whether intravenous thrombolysis or primary percutaneous coronary intervention is applied depends on local availability, organizational structures to achieve a short 'door-to-open-artery' time, the duration of symptoms and the presence of cardiogenic shock (Keeley et al., 2003).

9.2 Reperfusion adjunctive therapy in clinical practice

9.2.1 Standard medical therapy

Supplemental oxygen, in particular if blood oxygen saturation is below 90%, and adequate analgesia, using repeated doses of morphine sulphate, are standard measures in patients with AMI, which have been found to be useful in clinical practice; however evidence from large-scale randomized trials is lacking. Nitroglycerin may be administered for relief of anginal symptoms, pulmonary congestion or arterial hypertension, as long as systemic arterial blood pressure is sufficient (>100 mmHg systolic) and no right heart infarction is suspected. However, if arterial blood pressure is marginal, β-blocking agents, which may lower arterial blood pressure as well, should be used in preference due to their potential infarct size limiting effects (Antman et al., 2004).

9.2.2 Maintaining coronary artery patency

Administration of aspirin (initial oral dose 162–325 mg, then 75–162 mg daily) is standard treatment in AMI. Additional anti-platelet therapy with clopidogrel or ticlopidine was shown to be beneficial in STEMI not only for patients with coronary stent implantation. The CLARITY-TIMI 28-study demonstrated a significant reduction of re-infarction within 30 days after myocardial infarction in patients with clopidogrel as an adjunct to standard therapy and fibrinolysis (Sabatine et al., 2005). Administration of abciximab during primary angioplasty or maybe other glycoprotein IIb/IIIa receptor blockers, such as tirofiban or eptifibatide, started prior to PTCA, may result in higher rates of coronary artery patency, better preservation of contractile function and microvascular flow. Unfractionated heparin is standard therapy for patients undergoing percutaneous revascularisation, as an adjunct to fibrin-specific fibrinolytic agents (e.g. alteplase) and in patients at high risk for systemic thromboembolism such as large anterior myocardial infarctions, atrial

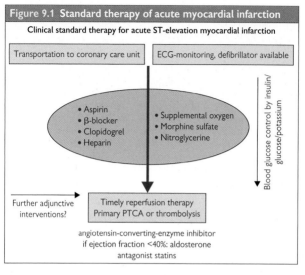

Figure 9.1 Standard therapy of acute myocardial infarction

Clinical standard therapy for acute ST-elevation myocardial infarction

Transportation to coronary care unit | ECG-monitoring, defibrillator available

- Aspirin
- β-blocker
- Clopidogrel
- Heparin

- Supplemental oxygen
- Morphine sulfate
- Nitroglycerine

Blood glucose control by insulin/ glucose/potassium

Further adjunctive interventions? → Timely reperfusion therapy Primary PTCA or thrombolysis

angiotensin-converting-enzyme inhibitor if ejection fraction <40%: aldosterone antagonist statins

fibrillation, or known intra-cardiac thrombus irrespective of the administered fibrinolytic drug. Several investigations suggested that low-molecular-weight heparin may be an alternative when dosing is adequately adjusted in renal insufficiency. The role of novel anticoagulation and antiplatelet agents, such as bivalirudin, and others, will be further defined in the next few years, but may be considered in special patients, e.g. in patients with known heparin-induced thrombocytopenia (type II) (Antman et al., 2004).

9.2.3 Adjunctive therapy to minimize energy demands during ischaemia

Energy expenditure during myocardial ischaemia is an important determinant of the resultant amount of myocardial necrosis. The administration of β-blocking agents, however, has become standard clinical treatment for all patients with acute myocardial infarction, provided that they are not compromised by cardiogenic shock and do not have relevant atrioventricular conduction disturbances or bradycardia. They reduce infarct size, the incidence of re-infarction and the frequency of ventricular tachyarrhythmias, and thereby may also be of benefit when reperfusion therapy is not successful. Administration as early as possible appears to be crucial for the maximum effectiveness (Robert et al., 1991).

9.2.4 **Adjunctive therapy to attenuate left ventricular remodelling**

Inhibitors of the renin-angiotensin-aldosterone system favourably influence the remodelling process of the left ventricle after the initial ischaemic insult. Within the first 24 hours an angiotensin-converting-enzyme inhibitor should be administered orally when arterial blood pressure is sufficient (>100 mHg systolic blood pressure). In particular, patients with anterior myocardial infarction, pulmonary congestion and left ventricular ejection fraction of less than 40% are expected to benefit. Angiotensin-receptor blockers are an alternative in patients intolerant to angiotensin-converting-enzyme inhibitors. During the first week, aldosterone receptor antagonists should also be started in patients with markedly reduced ejection fraction (Pitt et al., 2003).

9.3 **Adjunctive therapy targeting lethal reperfusion injury**

Many agents and concepts of adjunctive therapy applied during the early reperfusion period have been tested under clinical conditions in an attempt to attenuate the detrimental sequelae of myocardial reperfusion, as suggested from experimental research (Figure 9.2). Many of these clinical investigations were in part negative or not consistent so that no adjunctive therapy can be regarded as fully established for the treatment of reperfusion injury in the clinical setting. Reasons for the discrepancies compared with animal studies are varied (Yellon & Hausenloy, 2007). In some investigations, sub-group analyses suggested potentially relevant effects in specialized subsets of patients such as those with anterior myocardial infarction and early coronary artery reperfusion. The most important studies will be discussed in the following sections.

9.3.1 **Adenosine as reperfusion adjunctive therapy**

Experimental animal studies have clearly demonstrated that adenosine and adenosine receptor subtype-specific agonists confer powerful cardioprotection. Adenosine is able to mimic the cardioprotective effects of both ischaemic preconditioning and postconditioning and can inhibit platelet aggregation and reduce inflammation. In 1999, Mahaffey et al., (1999) published the first clinical study (AMISTAD) examining the role of adenosine as an adjunct to reperfusion in 236 patients presenting with STEMI. Patients who were randomized to 70 mcg/kg/min adenosine for 3 hours in combination with reperfusion therapy, experienced a significantly smaller myocardial infarct size (by 33%) as assessed by technetium-99m sestamibi SPECT. However, no difference in clinical endpoints was demonstrated. In the larger

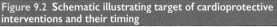

Figure 9.2 **Schematic illustrating target of cardioprotective interventions and their timing**

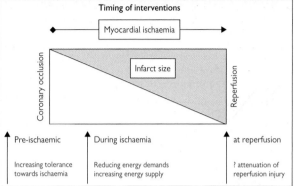

Timing of interventions

Myocardial ischaemia

Coronary occlusion

Infarct size

Reperfusion

Pre-ischaemic | During ischaemia | at reperfusion

Increasing tolerance towards ischaemia | Reducing energy demands increasing energy supply | ? attenuation of reperfusion injury

AMISTAD II study, in which 2,084 patients with acute anterior myocardial infarction were randomized to placebo, 50 mcg/kg/min or 70 mcg/kg/min adenosine in conjunction with reperfusion therapy, infarct size in the high-dose group (11% of the left ventricle) was significantly less than placebo (27% of the left ventricle) (Ross et al., 2005). However, again no difference in clinical endpoints could be demonstrated. A retrospective (post-hoc) subgroup analysis, calculated that only patients receiving reperfusion therapy within the first 3.17 hours after onset of symptoms demonstrated improved clinical outcome with adenosine therapy, while patients reperfused after this time did not significantly benefit from adenosine (Kloner et al., 2006).

9.3.2 **Anti-oxidants as reperfusion adjunctive therapy**

Early upon reperfusion, reactive oxygen species are generated by the enzyme xanthine oxidase, by cardiomyocyte mitochondria and by neutrophil NADPH oxidase, mediating functional myocardial reperfusion injury (stunning), chemoattraction of neutrophils and reduction of bioavailability of nitric oxide. While several animal studies have demonstrated cardioprotective effects by interventions reducing this 'oxygen paradox', most clinical studies have been inconclusive. For example, intravenous superoxide dismutase given prior to PCI for AMI, did not improve recovery of left ventricular contractile function, as assessed by contrast left ventriculography and radionuclide ventriculography within the first 24 hours and 4–6 weeks later (Flaherty et al., 1994). Similarly, the antioxidant trimetazidine, administered to patients with AMI in a large scale trial (19,725 patients, 56% with thrombolysis, 44% without thrombolysis) did not improve outcome (survival at 35 days and up to 3 years). However, in the subset of patients receiving thrombolysis, there was a non-significant trend towards increased mortality with trimetazidine treatment (EMIP-FR group, 2000). A single-centre study (101 patients), in which the oxygen radical scavenger edavarone was administered prior to primary angioplasty with stenting, demonstrated lower peak creatine-kinase levels, less arrhythmia and lower incidence of new Q-waves on ECG along with reduced cardiac events over approximately 3 years (Tsujita et al., 2006). However, overall event rate was very low in this study, in which reperfusion therapy was successful in all patients.

9.3.3 Glucose-insulin-potassium therapy

Several small clinical studies both in the pre-thrombolytic era and after the advent of thrombolysis have investigated the effects of an infusion of glucose/insulin/potassium (GIK) as an adjunct to reperfusion in patients presenting with an AMI. Most of these trials have demonstrated a trend towards or significantly less adverse cardiac events in patients on GIK therapy. In particular, diabetic patients appeared to benefit in the DIGAMI-trial (306 patients) (Malmberg et al., 1995). Of note, a subset of patients with heart failure demonstrated worse outcomes in the trial published by Von der Horst et al., (2003), while those without heart failure showed improved clinical outcome with GIK. The CREATE-ECLA trial, including 20,201 patients with AMI world-wide, however, did not show any significant difference in mortality, incidence of cardiac arrest, cardiogenic shock and re-infarction within 30 days for the entire study as well as for pre-defined subgroups (with or without reperfusion therapy, diabetic and non diabetic patients, with and without heart failure) (Mehta et al., 2005); however this trial therapy was associated with a high rate of hyperglycaemia. Another trial (IMMEDIATE trial) is still in progress in which early treatment with GIK therapy of patients with AMI will be investigated. Based on the currently available data, consequent control of blood glucose by intravenous insulin, potentially in combination with glucose, is recommended in patients with acute myocardial infarction, in particular diabetic patients, even if a clinically meaningful effect on infarct size has not been undoubtedly demonstrated.

9.3.4 Magnesium and calcium-antagonists

Administration of intravenous magnesium sulphate, which is known to have antiarrhythmic effects and which might serve as a mild calcium antagonist, as an adjunct to thrombolysis resulted in reduced mortality and heart failure in the early LIMIT-2 trial including 2,316 patients. However, subsequent studies (ISIS-4: 4,319 patients and MAGIC: 6,213 patients) failed to confirm these promising results both in combination with thrombolysis and primary angioplasty for acute myocardial infarction (reviewed in Yellon & Hausenloy, 2007).

In theory, myocardial calcium overload after ischaemia/reperfusion might be reduced by pharmacologic calcium antagonism. However, the calcium-antagonist, diltiazem, administered orally 1.5 to 4 days after onset of symptoms failed to reduce cardiac death and non-fatal re-infarction six months after thrombolysis in a trial including 874 patients; although the need for revascularisation was reduced with diltiazem treatment in this study (Boden *et al.*, 2000). Of note, patients with congestive heart failure were excluded from this study, as diltiazem (a non-dihydropyridine calcium antagonist) may have exacerbated heart failure. It is widely known that nifedipine, a short acting dihydropyridine-type calcium channel blocker, administered to patients with AMI increased mortality in another study, potentially due to reflex tachycardia. Therefore, calcium antagonists, in particular short-acting dihydropyridine-type calcium channel blockers, are generally not recommended in patients with AMI unless there is another indication such as hypertension (in which case long-acting dihydropyridine-agents should be used) or rapid atrioventricular conduction with atrial fibrillation (in which case non-dihydropyridine agents should be used when β-blockers are contra-indicated).

9.3.5 Na$^+$/H$^+$-exchange inhibitors

Attenuation of intracellular calcium overload appears to be the mechanism of cardioprotection conferred by Na$^+$/H$^+$-exchange inhibitors in experimental animal studies. An early clinical study, evaluating 100 patients with primary angioplasty for acute anterior myocardial infarction reported improved ejection fraction at 3 weeks, as assessed by serial contrast ventriculograms, and marginally reduced infarct size, as assessed by release of creatine-kinase isoform MB, in patients administered intravenous cariporide prior to primary angioplasty (Rupprecht *et al.*, 2000). However, ventriculograms were only considered to be sufficient for analysis in 55% of these patients which substantially weakened the results. The larger ESCAMI-trial (1,389 patients), which investigating eniporide as an adjunct to thrombolysis or primary PTCA, did not show beneficial effects on infarct size or clinical events (Zeymer *et al.*, 2001). This class of drugs has also been investigated in the setting of CABG surgery – see chapter 7).

9.3.6 **Anti-inflammatory agents**

Several anti-inflammatory agents with different targets have been tested in smaller and large scale clinical trials. These include, antibodies against CD-18, CD-11, P-selectin and complement factor C5, with the vast majority of these trials being negative. The largest trial (APEX AMI-trial: 5745 patients), testing pexelizumab, an antibody against C5-complement, as an adjunct to primary angioplasty for AMI, did not show a difference in 30 day mortality or 90 day incidence of death and heart failure (Armstrong *et al.*, 2007). Interestingly, the preceding COMMA trial had also failed to show reduction of infarct size with pexelizumab, however, 90-day mortality in this trial using primary PTCA as reperfusion strategy was significantly reduced with pexelizumab (Granger *et al.*, 2003).

9.3.7 **Nicorandil**

Nicorandil is a K_{ATP}-channel opening drug with nitrate-like action. It was investigated in several trials of stable coronary artery disease (e.g. IONA trial) where it demonstrated significant benefit in some combined end points. However, there were conflicting results for nicorandil as an adjunct to primary PTCA in acute myocardial infarction. The largest trial (J-WIND) did not show any beneficial effect on mortality, infarct size, and myocardial perfusion parameters (Kitakaze *et al.*, 2007).

9.3.8 **Atrial natriuretic peptide**

The multicentre placebo-controlled J-WIND trial also investigated whether an intravenous infusion of atrial natriuretic peptide for three days after reperfusion therapy could reduce infarct size and improve clinical outcome. In the 277 patients assigned to atrial natriuretic peptide infusion, infarct size, determined as creatine kinase release, was reduced by 14.7% and left ventricular ejection fraction was significantly improved at 6–12 months of follow-up in comparison to 292 placebo patients. Importantly, re-admission for heart failure and cardiac death rates were significantly reduced in patients receiving atrial natriuretic peptide (Kitakaze *et al.*, 2007). Therefore, infusion of atrial natriuretic peptide as an adjunct to reperfusion appears to be a promising approach which needs further investigation.

9.4 **Conclusions**

Parallel to the growing body of basic experimental research in the field of reperfusion injury, randomized, multi-center, placebo-controlled clinical studies will be required for every adjunctive intervention before it can be recommended for clinical routine. In particular, the reasons for the many discrepancies between basic animal research and clinical studies, undertaken to date, must be specified to increase the efficacy of scientific work. Table 9.1 lists some interventions tested in clinical trials or interventions currently under investigation. In addition to pharmacologic adjunctive therapy, non-pharmacologic interventions, such as ischaemic postconditioning (i.e. short reocclusions of the coronary artery after primary PTCA) or remote postconditioning (periods of ischaemia and reperfusion in remote organs during primary PTCA), need to be investigated in larger trials.

Table 9.1 Previous and ongoing attempts of pharmacological and non-pharmacological interventions targeting reperfusion

Intervention	Comment
β-blocking agents	Early administration may reduce infarct size, incidence of arrhythmia, mortality and infarct complications.
Atrial natriuretic peptide	The J-Wind trial demonstrated reduction of infarct size, improvement of left ventricular ejection fraction and prognostic benefit.
Adenosine, subtype specific adenosine agonists	Intravenous administration within 15 minutes of reperfusion (70 mcg/kg/min) may reduce infarct size. No clear prognostic benefit was shown for the entire study population, however, in the subgroup with early reperfusion, the combined endpoint of congestive heart failure and death rate at 6 months was reduced in the AMISTAD 2 trial.
Glucose-insulin-potassium-infusion (GIK therapy)	Intensive blood glucose control by insulin is recommended in diabetic patients; hyperglycaemia should be avoided. Caution is advisable in patients with cardiogenic shock or congestive heart failure. No benefit in CREATE-ECLA study.
Anti-oxidants (superoxide dismutase, trimetazidine, allopurinol, edavarone)	Most of the clinical studies have been negative. A smaller clinical trial using edavarone has showed some promise.
Anti-inflammation agents (pexelizumab, P-selectin antagonist, anti-CD 18 and anti CD 11 antibodies)	Clinical studies have been largely negative.
Alteration of cellular ion homeostasis (calcium antagonists, Na^+/H^+ exchange inhibitors)	In CABG surgery, the incidence of myocardial infarction may be reduced with Na^+/H^+-exchange inhibition. Larger trials in acute myocardial infarction were negative. Stroke and renal failure were unexpected side effects in some studies. Studies using calcium-antagonists were mostly negative.
Magnesium	Magnesium infusion reduced infarct size and incidence of heart failure in the LIMIT-2 trial. Subsequent large scale trials, however, have been negative.
Nicorandil, potassium channel openers	As an adjunct to reperfusion therapy, no benefit on clinical outcomes was demonstrated.

Key references

Antman, E.M., Anbe, D.T., Armstrong, P.W., et al., (2004). American College of Cardiology; American Heart Association Task Force on Practice Guidelines; Canadian Cardiovascular Society. ACC/AHA guidelines for the management of patients with ST-elevation myocardial infarction: a report of the American College of Cardiology/American Heart Association Task Force on Practice Guidelines (Committee to Revise the 1999 Guidelines for the Management of Patients with Acute Myocardial Infarction). Circulation, 110: 588–636.

Armstrong, P.W., Granger, C.B., Adams, P.X., et al., (2007). APEX AMI Investigators. Pexelizumab for acute ST-elevation myocardial infarction in patients undergoing primary percutaneous coronary intervention: a randomized controlled trial. JAMA, 297: 43–51.

Boden, W.E., van Gilst, W.H., Scheldewaert, R.G., et al., (2000). Diltiazem in acute myocardial infarction treated with thrombolytic agents: a randomized placebo-controlled trial. Incomplete Infarction Trial of European Research Collaborators Evaluation Prognosis post-Thrombolysis (INTERCEPT). Lancet, 355: 1751–1756.

EMIP-FR group. (2000). Effect of 48-h intravenous trimetazidine on short- and long-term outcomes of patients with acute myocardial infarction, with and without thrombolytic therapy; A double-blind, placebo-controlled, randomized trial. The EMIP-FR Group. European Myocardial Infarction Project–Free Radicals. Eur Heart J, 21: 1537–1546.

Flaherty, J.T., Pitt, B., Gruber, J.W., et al., (1994). Recombinant human superoxide dismutase (h-SOD) fails to improve recovery of ventricular function in patients undergoing coronary angioplasty for acute myocardial infarction. Circulation, 89: 1982–1991.

Granger, C.B., Mahaffey, K.W., Weaver, W.D., et al., (2003). Pexelizumab, an anti-C5 complement antibody, as an adjunctive therapy to primary percutaneous coronary intervention in acute myocardial infarction: the COMplement inhibition in Myocardial infarction treated with Angioplasty (COMMA) trial. Circulation, 108: 1184–1190.

Keeley, E.C., Boura, J.A., and Grines, C.L. (2003). Primary angioplasty versus intravenous thrombolytic therapy for acute myocardial infarction: a quantitative review of 23 randomized trials. Lancet, 361: 13–20.

Kitakaze, M., Asakura, M., Shintani, Y., et al., (2007). Human atrial natriuretic peptide and nicorandil as adjuncts to reperfusion treatment for acute myocardial infarction (J-WIND): two randomized trials. Lancet, 370: 1483–1493.

Kloner, R.A., Forman, M.B., Gibbons, R.J., et al., (2006). Impact of time to therapy and reperfusion modality on the efficacy of adenosine in acute myocardial infarction: the AMISTAD-2 trial. Eur. Heart J, 27: 2400–2405.

Mahaffey, K.W., Puma, J.A., Barbagelata, N.A., et al., (1999). Adenosine as an adjunct to thrombolytic therapy for acute myocardial infarction: results of a multicenter, randomized, placebo-controlled trial: the Acute Myocardial Infarction STudy of ADenosine (AMISTAD) trial. J Am Coll Cardiol, 34: 1711–1720.

Malmberg, K., Rydén, L., Efendic, S., *et al.*, (1995). Randomized trial of insulin-glucose infusion followed by subcutaneous insulin treatment in diabetic patients with acute myocardial infarction (DIGAMI study): effects on mortality at 1 year. *J Am Coll Cardiol.* **26**: 57–65.

Mehta, S.R., Yusuf, S., Díaz, R., *et al.*, (2005). CREATE-ECLA Trial Group Investigators. Effect of glucose-insulin-potassium infusion on mortality in patients with acute ST-segment elevation myocardial infarction: the CREATE-ECLA randomized controlled trial. *JAMA*, **293**: 437–446.

Pitt, B., Remme, W., Zannad, F., Neaton, J., *et al.*, (2003). Eplerenone post-acute myocardial infarction heart failure efficacy and survival study investigators. Eplerenone, a selective aldosterone blocker, in patients with left ventricular dysfunction after myocardial infarction. *N Engl J Med*, **348**: 1309–1321.

Roberts, R., Rogers, W.J., Mueller, H.S., *et al.*, (1991). Immediate versus deferred beta-blockade following thrombolytic therapy in patients with acute myocardial infarction: results of the Thrombolysis in Myocardial Infarction (TIMI) II-B study. *Circulation*, **83**: 422–437.

Ross, A.M., Gibbon, R.J., Stone, G.W., *et al.*, (2005). A randomized, double-blinded, placebo-controlled multicenter trial of adenosine as an adjunct to reperfusion in the treatment of acute myocardial infarction (AMISTAD-II). *J Am Coll Cardiol*, **45**: 1775–1780.

Rupprecht, H.J., vom Dahl, J., Terres, W., *et al.*, (2000). Cardioprotective effects of the Na^+/H^+ exchange inhibitor cariporide in patients with acute anterior myocardial infarction undergoing direct PTCA. *Circulation*, **101**: 2902–2908.

Sabatine, M.S., Cannon, C.P., Gibson, C.M., *et al.*, (2005). CLARITY TIMI 28 Investigators. Addition of clopidogrel to aspirin and fibrinolytic therapy for myocardial infarction with ST-segment elevation. *N Engl J Med*, **352**: 1179–1189.

Tsujita, K., Shimomura, H., Kaita, K., *et al.*, (2006). Long-term efficacy of edavarone in patients with acute myocardial infarction. *Circ J*, **70**: 832–837.

Von Der Horst, I.C., Zijlstra, F., van't Hof, A.W., *et al.*, (2003). Zwolle Infarct Study Group. Glucose-insulin-potassium infusion in patients treated with primary angioplasty for acute myocardial infarction: the glucose-insulin-potassium study: a randomized trial. *J Am Coll Cardiol*, **42**: 784–791.

Yellon, D., and Hausenloy, D. (2007). Mechanism of disease: myocardial reperfusion injury. *N Engl J Med*, **357**: 1121–1135.

Zeymer, U., Suryapranata, H., Monassier, J.P., *et al.*, (2001). ESCAMI Investigators. The Na^+/H^+ exchange inhibitor eniporide as an adjunct to early reperfusion therapy for acute myocardial infarction: results of the evaluation of the safety and cardioprotective effects of eniporide in acute myocardial infarction (ESCAMI) *J Am Coll Cardiol*, **38**: 1644–1650.

Chapter 10

Stem Cell Therapy Post-AMI

Philippe Menasché

Key points

- Experimental studies suggest that bone marrow-derived stem cells can improve function of infarcted myocardium
- This benefit seems to involve paracrine signalling and limitation of left ventricular remodelling rather than true regeneration of cardiomyocytes from donor cells
- These experimental findings have been translated in the clinical setting into significant, although moderate, improvements in cardiac function and LV remodelling but the extent to which these benefits impact on event-free long term survival remains to be determined
- Optimisation of this therapeutic strategy will require a more comprehensive characterisation of cell functionality and an improvement in the methods used in cell transfer, engraftment, survival and integration.

10.1 Introduction

Regenerative therapy using stem cells is currently generating an escalating interest as a potential treatment option in patients presenting with an acute myocardial infarction (AMI) and in patients with chronic heart failure. In the former setting, the seminal publication by Orlic *et al.*, (2001) first raised the possibility that bone marrow-derived cells may engraft into acutely ischaemic myocardium and improve left ventricular (LV) function. Although these studies were performed in mice models according to protocols of questionable relevance, they immediately triggered a series of phase I human trials that have invariably reported 'positive' results and contributed to an excessive hype that has been somewhat dampened by the subsequently reported outcomes of more rigorously conducted randomized controlled trials. It may now be the appropriate time to review this burgeoning field of research and to realistically outline the hurdles that need to be overcome before we can claim that the regeneration of acutely infarcted myocardium can really be achieved and positively affect event-free long-term survival.

10.2 **Is there an unmet clinical need?**

Over the past decades, the treatment of acute myocardial infarction has dramatically improved, largely because of the extensive use of thrombolysis or balloon-based coronary interventions targeted at early reperfusion of the culprit coronary artery. However, it is estimated that still up to one-third of eligible patients with ST-segment elevation acute myocardial infarction (STEMI) do not receive reperfusion therapy acutely (Boden *et al.*, 2007).

Thus, there still remains a significant proportion of patients who might benefit from additional treatments designed, at best to promote myocardial regeneration and at the very least to limit LV remodelling. Several criteria primarily derived from echocardiography and delayed gadolinium-enhancement magnetic resonance imaging have now been shown to be predictive of late remodelling. These include microvas-cular obstruction and infarct size, factors which are clinically relevant given that interventions known to slow or revert remodelling are associated with improved clinical outcomes (Cioffi *et al.*, 2005). Taken together, these findings can be used to stratify subsets of patients which are more likely to benefit from adjunctive therapies like cell transplantation.

10.3 **What are the clinical results?**

10.3.1 **Types of infused cells**

Until now, only three types of cells have undergone clinical testing in the setting of a ST-elevation myocardial infarction (STEMI):

1. mononuclear cells (MNC) derived from either bone marrow or peripheral blood;
2. CD133$^+$ progenitors; and
3. mesenchymal stem cells (MSC).

Mononuclear cells

Most studies have focused on MNC extemporaneously processed from bone marrow aspirates of the pelvic crest and re-injected into the infarct-related artery a few days after its recanalization by balloon angioplasty and stenting. On the basis of a recent meta-analysis that has compiled the results of 10 randomized controlled trials comprising 698 patients (Lipinski *et al.*, 2007), bone marrow cell transplantation improved LV ejection fraction by 3.0% and reduced both infarct size and LV end-systolic volume by 5.6% and 7.4 ml, respectively (all these differences being statistically significant compared with controls).

The safety of the procedure was also established by this review. However, these efficacy data should be interpreted with caution because of several limitations including the small sample size of each tabulated study, their short follow-up (median time of 6 months), the potentially confounding role of additional cytokine-induced bone marrow cell mobilization or the use of $CD133^+$ progenitors, the inconsistent blinding of involved caregivers and, overall, the huge variability in application schedules and cell dosing.

By restricting the analysis of outcomes to the four major randomized controlled trials of intracoronary MNC infusions, we are left with only one trial (the 204-patient REPAIR-AMI study) which has actually met its primary end point by showing a significant increase in angiographically-measured ejection fraction up to 12 months in treated patients compared with placebo-infused controls (Schächinger et al., 2006). This increase, however, represented an absolute change in ejection fraction of only 2.5%. In contrast, the other three major randomized trials (Wollert et al., 2004; Janssens et al., 2006; Lunde et al., 2006) failed to meet their primary end point (LV ejection fraction) even though one of them (Janssens et al., 2006) provided encouraging hints with regard to a reduction in infarct size measured by MRI. Furthermore, the benefits of intracoronary infusions of MNC reported at 4 months in the BOOST trial (Wollert et al., 2004) were no longer apparent 14 months later because of a gradual improvement in the control group (Meyer et al., 2006).

The explanation for these discordant results remains unclear but are not really surprising if one takes into consideration the differences in patient- and cell-related factors. The role of these confounding factors is clearly illustrated by the identification, in the REPAIR-MI trial, of pre-procedural LV function, pro-NT-BNP serum levels, cell functionality and the timing of therapy as predictive factors of outcome (Schächinger et al., 2006; Assmus et al., 2007).

A strong argument made by the REPAIR-MI investigators to explain the discrepancy between their positive results and the totally negative ones of the ASTAMI trial is that, differences in cell preparation may profoundly affect graft functionality (Seeger et al., 2007a). The ASTAMI trial investigators have replied that the positive results in REPAIR-MI might conversely have been driven by the relatively poor outcome seen in the placebo group, possibly because of some toxicity of the control medium (Arnesen et al., 2007). The accuracy of single-plane angiocardiography for assessing LV function and volumes in the REPAIR-MI trial has also been challenged and indeed the magnitude of the increase in ejection fraction seen in the cell-treated group of this trial is similar to the MRI-derived values reported following primary percutaneous intervention after STEMI in the absence of any cell therapy (Ripa et al., 2006).

CD133$^+$ progenitors

Using a similar intracoronary route of cell transfer, other investigators have focused on the specific population of CD133$^+$ progenitors (Mansour et al., 2006). However, despite some evidence for improvement in LV function, they stopped the trial prematurely because of the worrisome observation of a higher-than-expected rate of in-stent restenosis. Whether these findings reflect the Janus phenomenon whereby the downside effect of pro-angiogenic cells is to also stimulate atherogenesis or are only due to bad luck in a small group of patients remains currently uncertain. It is clear, however, that additional mechanistic insights are required before the intracoronary application of this cell population can be safely recommended for clinical applications.

Mesenchymal stem cells

Mesenchymal stem cells comprise the third cell type which has been investigated. In the randomized placebo-controlled trial conducted by Chen et al., (2004), LV function and perfusion were found to be significantly improved three months after the procedure in treated patients compared with those infused with saline but so far, these results have not been duplicated. Indeed, a major advantage of MSC is their alleged immune privilege that could allow their potential use as an allogeneic off-the-shelf readily available cell therapy product. This immediate availability is a clear advantage when therapy is required in an acute setting and a company-sponsored randomized controlled double-blind trial (Provacel™ study) has recently tested this concept by assessing the effects of injecting intravenously allogeneic MSC in patients with STEMI. Six months later, LV function was found to be significantly improved compared with baseline values in treated patients but these outcome measurements did not differ significantly from those obtained in control patients. The latter result highlights the major problem of the optimal route for MSC delivery. Thus, intracoronary infusions, as used in the study of Chen et al., (2004) raise a safety concern related to distal capillary plugging due to the large size of MSC and subsequent microinfarctions whereas systemic intravenous infusion, which is obviously much safer, is unlikely to be functionally effective because extracardiac trapping of MSC prevents them to substantially home in the target myocardium (Freyman et al., 2006). As for the direct intramyocardial transfer of MSC which is more relevant to chronic clinical settings, it seems to be fraught with a potential risk of calcification (Breitbach et al., 2007). Additional studies are thus warranted to better characterise the mechanisms of the immune tolerance to MSC and determine which route, if any, could allow their safe and effective delivery to the myocardium.

10.3.2 **Other approaches**

Aside from the direct intracoronary infusion of bone marrow-derived cells, the assumption that their intramyocardial engraftment could contribute to the repair of infarcted tissue has led to an alternate strategy based on cytokine-induced mobilization by using granulocyte colony-stimulating factor (G-CSF) to increase the circulating pool of progenitors and enhance their subsequent homing in sites of injury. So far, the safety profile of G-CSF treatment has been rather reassuring (Ince et al., 2007). However, three randomized controlled trials have failed to show any benefit on function, perfusion or infarct size, regardless of whether the drug was given in patients undergoing early (Valgimigli et al., 2005; Zohlnhöfer et al., 2006; Ripa et al., 2006) or delayed (Engelmann et al., 2006) reperfusion and the only 'positive' study (Ince et al., 2005) had not included true controls. Put together, these data indicate that there is currently no evidence that G-CSF provides any additional benefit over best-of-care management of patients with acute myocardial infarction.

10.4 **Possible cardioprotective mechanisms underlying stem cell therapy**

10.4.1 **Stem cells and myocardial regeneration**

Regeneration implies the formation of new cardiomyocytes that can be either donor- or host-derived. So far, there is no conclusive evidence that bone marrow cells actually undergo a true cardiomyogenic differentiation (Murry et al., 2004), and it is now increasingly recognised that most of the previously reported transdifferentiation patterns were in fact immunofluorescence-associated artefacts or fusion events. The only animal study that has most closely mimicked the clinical scenario has been reported by Moelker et al., (2006). Using a swine model of reperfused myocardial infarction, these authors have injected total bone marrow cells or its MNC fraction into the reopened coronary artery and assessed the outcomes one month later by MRI. Their results failed to document any benefit of infused cells on ejection fraction or LV volumes or any evidence for a cardiomyogenic differentiation of the grafted cells although they showed a reduction in infarct size that closely duplicated the clinical data of Janssens et al., (2006). Interestingly, this animal study has lagged behind the initial clinical trials by 5 years as most of the preceding laboratory experiments had used animal models and cell delivery protocols of questionable clinical relevance. This unusual absence of streamlined bench to bedside transition and its major consequence, i.e., a flurry of human trials lacking a robust preclinical foundation, has unfortunately contributed to cloud the entire field and to generate confusion among patients, caregivers and regulators.

Indeed, among bone marrow cells, the mesenchymal fraction is the one which has the greatest propensity to differentiate along the mesodermal lineage but even though they express cardiac markers, there is still no evidence that once engrafted, they develop an active-force generating capacity and form a functional syncytium contributing to augment pump function. The alternate hypothesis is that the infused cells release mediators that could 'awake' cardiac stem cells harboured in quiescent niches (Smith et al., 2007) and drive them towards differentiation into more mature cardiomyocytes with an attendant improvement in LV function. However, the applicability of these findings to the human adult ischaemic myocardium remains uncertain.

10.4.2 **Stem cells and LV remodelling**

One of the most serious complications of an acute myocardial infarction is the progressive development of LV remodelling which then leads to heart failure. Experimentally, there are some arguments supporting the hypothesis that stem cells could beneficially interfere with this process. This could occur through a mechanical increase in scar thickness by packed cells and/or the cell-derived release of cytokines causing changes in the composition of the extracellular matrix which, in turn, would translate into decreased fibrosis and increased scar elasticity. Put together, these mechanisms may account for several experimental observations that cell transplantation limits remodelling. However, this finding has not been corroborated by the results of the above mentioned meta-analysis which have failed to show a significant decrease in LV end-diastolic volumes in cell-treated patients.

10.4.3 **Stem cells and paracrine signalling**

Considering that only a tiny fraction of the bone marrow cells infused by the intracoronary route can gain access to myocardial tissue and that most of the initially engrafted cells then rapidly die (see below), the most likely mechanism of action is the paracrine activation of signalling pathways leading primarily to increased angiogenesis and limitation of apoptosis. This hypothesis is largely supported by the finding that bone marrow cells secrete angiogenic cytokines (Kinnaird et al., 2004) and survival factors like Akt (Gnecchi et al., 2006). Altogether, these soluble mediators could explain the MNC-related reduction in infarct size reported in Moelker's study (2006) and confirmed by the meta-analysis (Lipinski et al., 2007). It is thus noteworthy that stem cells might improve heart function by mechanisms (such as paracrine signaling and increasing scar thickness which would be expected to reduce wall stress on remote myocardium) that are distinct from the generation of newly formed donor-derived contractile units.

10.5 What are the remaining hurdles?

10.5.1 Cell type

At the acute stage of a myocardial infarction, the most stringent practical constraint is the immediate availability of the cell product to allow prompt institution of therapy. Bone marrow MNC fulfill this condition since they can be processed extemporaneously by density gradient centrifugation or only cultured for a few hours if the objective is to grow endothelial progenitors. Hematopoietic $CD34^+$ or $CD133^+$ progenitors can also be sorted from bone marrow aspirates; however, since time may be lacking for a cytokine-induced mobilization (which usually takes 5 days) followed by apheresis, the ultimate yield is expected to be quantitatively low since these progenitors represent approximately 1–2% of bone marrow cells. Bone marrow-derived mesenchymal cells are also attractive candidates in an acute situation because of their above mentioned immune privilege compatible with an allogeneic use. An alternate option is to isolate MSC extemporaneously from fat tissue by using a dedicated device. This approach is currently being tested clinically. Conversely, skeletal myoblasts are excluded from the onset because of the time required for expanding the muscle biopsy (2 to 3 weeks). Although this concern is not relevant to cord blood-derived stem cells which could be used, like MSC, as an allogeneic off-the-shelf product, these cells should probably be also discarded because their large size may cause distal capillary plugging and microinfarctions following an intracoronary infusion (Moelker et al., 2007). As for cardiac-specified human embryonic stem cells, their ability to generate cardiomyocytes (Tomescot et al., 2007) may make them more suitable for remuscularisation of chronic scars at a more remote time point after the index event.

Beyond the choice of a given type of cells, another fundamental, and yet unsettled issue, is to choose between autologous and allogeneic cells. Autologous cells have obvious advantages such as availability and lack of immunogenicity. However, with accumulating experience, their limitations are now also recognized. These include:

1. the large individual variability between patients;
2. the baseline impairment of bone marrow cell function in patients with ischaemic heart disease and
3. the cost of customized quality controls which need to be repeated for each patient-specific batch.

These hurdles are overcome by the use of an allogeneic cell product which can be prepared, tested and standardized beforehand but, in turn, raises the problem of its immunogenicity (except, maybe, in the case of MSC). Even though this limitation might be circumvented in the future by new and less aggressive immunosuppressive regimens, additional studies are warranted to thoroughly compare the risk-benefit and cost-effectiveness ratios of autologous versus allogeneic cell therapy products.

10.5.2 Modalities of cell delivery

The optimal technique of cell processing, dosing and timing of delivery still needs to be fine-tuned. Although the clinical outcome has been linked to cell function rather than to cell number, it would be desirable to have an estimate of the dose range required for achieving a successful result (in the meta-analysis of randomized trials reported above (Lipinski et al., 2007), the dose of MNC has ranged from 46×10^6 to $2,460 \times 10^6$ MNC). Interestingly, this meta-analysis showed a strong trend towards an association between injected volume (not cell number) and change in ejection fraction. Likewise, the optimal timing remains uncertain. Too early and a cell infusion may increase graft death because of the hostile inflammatory milieu, as suggested by the REPAIR-MI data showing maximal benefits when cells were given beyond 5 days after infarction. Conversely, too late and the infusions may have limited efficacy because of the loss of the appropriate signals. Clearly, additional experimental work is necessary to better define the most appropriate time window for stem cell therapy.

10.5.3 Enhancement of homing

A unique feature of acute myocardial infarction is that stem cells can only be delivered by intracoronary infusion in the reopened infarct-related artery. Whereas chronic angina or heart failure can benefit from surgical epicardial or catheter-based endoventricular cell injections. Clearly, these transfer techniques are not applicable to patients presenting with a STEMI, which would preclude any procedure requiring the puncture of freshly ischaemic endocardium. Although the intracoronary route of infusion has the advantage to be standardized and reproducible, its drawback is that despite an allegedly increased permeability of the ischaemic endothelium and the attraction of CXCR4-bearing circulating bone marrow cells by their ligand, stromal cell-derived factor 1 (SDF-1), only a small percentage of the infused cells can gain access to the myocardial tissue (only 1.3% to 2.6% of MNC, as assessed by positron emission tomography imaging in patients). This percentage dramatically increases (14%–39%) when the injected sample consists of selected $CD34^+$ cells (Hofmann et al., 2005) but, as shown above, the use of progenitors may be associated with safety issues. Finally, retrograde infusion of cells through the coronary sinus might be an attractive alternative for ensuring graft delivery (Yokohama et al., 2006) but it is more technically challenging, which could limit its clinical implementation.

Given the limited amount of infused cells successfully delivered to the myocardial interstitium by the intracoronary route, several pharmacological or physical strategies are currently under investigation to enhance their homing, engraftment and integration through priming of donor cells or manipulation of the host microenvironment to make it more permissive to grafted cells (Seeger *et al.*, 2007b). With all things considered, the best approach will be the one combining safety, preclinical efficacy, practicality of clinical implementation and regulatory approvability. In parallel, the development of these strategies requires an improvement in cell tracking techniques allowing a meaningful assessment of engraftment rates (Stuckey *et al.*, 2006).

10.6 Conclusions

Currently available data strongly suggest that some subsets of patients with STEMI might benefit from stem cell injections as an adjunctive therapy. This benefit, however, may not be necessarily mediated by a true regeneration of the infarcted myocardium and could involve salvage of jeopardized tissue by alternate mechanisms like paracrine signalling or limitation of late LV remodelling. Nevertheless, some important hurdles, particularly pertaining to variability of cell functionality, cell transfer, engraftment, survival and integration still need to be overcome before expectations raised by stem cell therapy can be converted into a clinically meaningful reality.

Key references

Arnesen, H., Lunde, K., Aakhus, S., *et al.*, (2007). Cell therapy in myocardial infarction. *Lancet*, **369**: 2142–2143.

Assmus, B., Fischer-Rasokat, U., Honold, J., *et al.*, (2007). TOPCARE-CHD Registry. Transcoronary transplantation of functionally competent BMCs is associated with a decrease in natriuretic peptide serum levels and improved survival of patients with chronic postinfarction heart failure: results of the TOPCARE-CHD Registry. *Circ Res*, **100**: 1234–1241.

Boden, W.E., Eagle, K., Granger, C.B. (2007). Reperfusion strategies in acute ST-segment elevation myocardial infarction: a comprehensive review of contemporary management options. *J Am Coll Cardiol*, **50**: 917–929.

Breitbach, M., Bostani, T., Roell, W., *et al.*, (2007). Potential risks of bone marrow cell transplantation into infarcted hearts. *Blood*, **110**: 1362–1369.

Cioffi, G., Tarantini, L., De Feo, S., *et al.*, (2005). Pharmacological left ventricular reverse remodeling in elderly patients receiving optimal therapy for chronic heart failure. *Eur J Heart Fail*, **7**: 1040–1048.

Chen, S.L., Fang, W.W., Ye, F., et al., (2004). Effect on left ventricular function of intracoronary transplantation of autologous bone marrow mesenchymal stem cell in patients with acute myocardial infarction. Am J Cardiol., **94**: 92–95.

Engelmann, M.G., Theiss, H.D., Hennig-Theiss, C., et al., (2006). Autologous bone marrow stem cell mobilization induced by granulocyte colony-stimulating factor after subacute ST-segment elevation myocardial infarction undergoing late revascularization: final results from the G-CSF-STEMI (Granulocyte Colony-Stimulating Factor ST-Segment Elevation Myocardial Infarction) trial. J Am Coll Cardiol, **48**: 1712–1721.

Freyman, T., Polin, G., Osman, H., et al., (2006). A quantitative, randomized study evaluating three methods of mesenchymal stem cell delivery following myocardial infarction. Eur Heart J, **27**: 1114–1122.

Gnecchi, M., He, H., Liang, O.D., et al., (2006). Evidence supporting paracrine hypothesis for Akt-modified mesenchymal stem cell-mediated cardiac protection and functional improvement. FASEB J, **20**: 661–669.

Hofmann, M., Wollert, K.C., Meyer, G.P., et al., (2005). Monitoring of bone marrow cell homing into the infarcted human myocardium. Circulation, **111**: 2198–2202.

Ince, H., Petzsch, M., Kleine, H.D., et al., (2005). Preservation from left ventricular remodeling by front-integrated revascularization and stem cell liberation in evolving acute myocardial infarction by use of granulocyte-colony-stimulating factor (FIRSTLINE-AMI). Circulation, **112**: 3097–3106.

Ince, H., Valgimigli, M., Petzsch, M., et al., (2007). Cardiovascular events and restenosis following administration of G-CSF in acute myocardial infarction: Systematic review of the literature and individual patient-data meta-analysis. Heart, Aug 29 (EPub).

Janssens, S., Dubois, C., Bogaert, J., et al., (2006). Autologous bone marrow-derived stem-cell transfer in patients with ST-segment elevation myocardial infarction: double-blind, randomized controlled trial. Lancet, **367**: 113–121.

Kinnaird, T., Stabile, E., Burnett, M.S., et al., (2004). Marrow-derived stromal cells express genes encoding a broad spectrum of arteriogenic cytokines and promote in vitro and in vivo arteriogenesis through paracrine mechanisms. Circ Res, **94**: 678–685.

Lipinski, M.J., Biondi-Zoccai, G., Abbate, A., et al., (2007). Impact of intra-coronary cell therapy on left ventricular function in the setting of acute myocardial infarction. J Am Coll Cardiol, **50**: 1761–1767.

Lunde, K., Solheim, S., Aakhus, S., et al., (2006). Intracoronary injection of mononuclear bone marrow cells in acute myocardial infarction. N Engl J Med, **355**: 1199–1209.

Mansour, S., Vanderheyden, M., De Bruyne, B., et al., (2006). Intracoronary delivery of hematopoietic bone marrow stem cells and luminal loss of the infarct-related artery in patients with recent myocardial infarction. J Am Coll Cardiol, **47**: 1727–1730.

Meyer, G.P., Wollert, K.C., Lotz, J., et al., (2006). Intracoronary bone marrow cell transfer after myocardial infarction: eighteen months' follow-up data from the randomized, controlled BOOST (BOne marrow transfer to enhance ST-elevation infarct regeneration) trial. *Circulation*, **113**: 1287–1294.

Moelker, A.D., Baks, T., van den Bos, E.J., et al., (2006). Reduction in infarct size, but no functional improvement after bone marrow cell administration in a porcine model of reperfused myocardial infarction. *Eur Heart J*, **27**: 3057–3064.

Moelker, A.D., Baks, T., Wever, K.M., et al., (2007). Intracoronary delivery of umbilical cord blood derived unrestricted somatic stem cells is not suitable to improve LV function after myocardial infarction in swine. *J Mol Cell Cardiol*, **42**: 735–745.

Murry, C.E., Soonpaa, M.H., Reinecke, H., et al., (2004). Haematopoietic stem cells do not transdifferentiate into cardiac myocytes in myocardial infarcts. *Nature*, **428**: 664–668.

Orlic, D., Kajstura, J., Chimenti, S., et al., (2001). Mobilized bone marrow cells repair the infarcted heart, improving function and survival. Proc *Natl Acad Sci U S A*, **98**: 10344–10349.

Ripa, R.S., Jorgensen, E., Wang, Y., et al., (2006). Stem cell mobilization induced by subcutaneous granulocyte-colony stimulating factor to improve cardiac regeneration after acute ST-elevation myocardial infarction: result of the double-blind, randomized, placebo-controlled stem cells in myocardial infarction (STEMMI) trial. *Circulation*, **113**: 1983–1992.

Schachinger, V., Erbs, S., Elsasser, A., et al., (2006). REPAIR-AMI Investigators. Intracoronary bone marrow-derived progenitor cells in acute myocardial infarction. *N Engl J Med*, **355**: 1210–1221.

Seeger, F.H., Tonn, T., Krzossok, N., et al., (2007a). Cell isolation procedures matter: a comparison of different isolation protocols of bone marrow mononuclear cells used for cell therapy in patients with acute myocardial infarction. *Eur Heart J*, **28**: 766–772.

Seeger, F.H., Zeiher, A.M., Dimmeler, S. (2007b). Cell-enhancement strategies for the treatment of ischemic heart disease. *Nat Clin Pract Cardiovasc Med., Suppl* **1**: S110–113.

Smith, R.R., Barile, L., Cho, H.C., et al., (2007). Regenerative potential of cardiosphere-derived cells expanded from percutaneous endomyocardial biopsy specimens. *Circulation*, **115**: 896–908.

Stuckey, D.J., Carr, C.A., Martin-Rendon, E., et al., (2006). Iron particles for noninvasive monitoring of bone marrow stromal cell engraftment into, and isolation of viable engrafted donor cells from, the heart. *Stem Cells*, **24**: 1968–1975.

Tomescot, A., Leschik, J., Bellamy, V., et al., (2007). Differentiation *in vivo* of cardiac committed human embryonic stem cells in postmyocardial infarcted rats. *Stem Cells.*, **25**: 2200–2205.

Valgimigli, M., Rigolin, G.M., Cittanti, C., et al., (2005). Use of granulocyte-colony stimulating factor during acute myocardial infarction to enhance bone marrow stem cell mobilization in humans: clinical and angiographic safety profile. *Eur Heart J*, **26**: 1838–1845.

Wollert, K.C., Meyer, G.P., Lotz, J., *et al.,* (2004). Intracoronary autologous bone-marrow cell transfer after myocardial infarction: the BOOST randomized controlled clinical trial. *Lancet,* **364**: 141–148.

Yokoyama, S., Fukuda, N., Li, Y., *et al.,* (2006). A strategy of retrograde injection of bone marrow mononuclear cells into the myocardium for the treatment of ischemic heart disease. *J Mol Cell Cardiol,* **40**: 24–34.

Zohlnhofer, D., Ott, I., Mehilli, J., *et al.,* (2006). REVIVAL-2 Investigators. Stem cell mobilization by granulocyte colony-stimulating factor in patients with acute myocardial infarction: a randomized controlled trial. *JAMA,* **95**: 1003–1010.

Chapter 11

Novel Cardioprotective Strategies

Derek Hausenloy & Derek Yellon

Key points

- Despite optimal therapy, the mortality and morbidity of coronary heart disease remains significant. Hence, novel treatment strategies of cardioprotection are required to improve clinical outcomes in these patients
- Experimental studies have provided a plethora of therapeutic strategies for reducing myocardial injury, but the translation of these findings into the clinical setting has been largely disappointing. Many of these unsuccessful clinical studies have relied upon individually targeting established mediators of lethal reperfusion injury such as oxidative stress, inflammation, calcium overload and so forth
- Clearly, novel targets for cardioprotection as well as a multi-targeted approach to cardioprotection directed against the multiple causes of lethal reperfusion injury are required to effect benefits in clinical outcomes
- In this regard, the introduction of ischaemic post-conditioning, a novel treatment strategy, in which following primary PCI the process of myocardial reperfusion is interrupted by several coronary re-occlusions, has been reported to reduce myocardial myocardial injury in AMI patients
- Furthermore, experimental studies have identified the Reperfusion Injury Salvage Kinase (RISK) pathway and the mitochondrial permeability transition pore (mPTP) as novel targets for cardioprotection, which are currently been examined in the clinical setting.

113

11.1 Need for novel cardioprotective strategies

Despite optimal therapy the mortality and morbidity from coronary artery disease in all its manifestations remains significant. The previous chapters have outlined what is considered optimal therapy in the setting of an acute myocardial infarction. These include the method of reperfusion, anti-platelet therapy, antithrombotic therapy and other medical therapy such as beta-blockers, ACE-inhibitors and 'statins'. Numerous attempts, with inconsistent results, have been made to further limit myocardial reperfusion injury in ST-elevation MI (STEMI) patients, and emerging strategies such as stem-cell therapy are currently being examined. However, novel and effective cardioprotective strategies are still required to reduce the extent of myocardial injury sustained in these different clinical settings in order to improve clinical outcomes. Several promising novel cardioprotective strategies are examined in this chapter (see Figure 11.1).

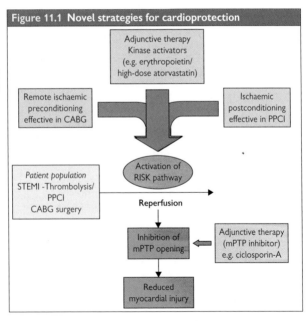

Figure 11.1 Novel strategies for cardioprotection

11.2 Ischaemic postconditioning

For patients presenting with an ST-elevation myocardial infarction (STEMI), the recently described interventional strategy of ischaemic postconditioning promises to be a potential novel effective cardio-protective strategy. Ischaemic postconditioning (IPost) refers to the cardioprotection obtained from interrupting myocardial reperfusion with three or more short-lived episodes (duration 30–60 sec) of myocardial ischaemia and reperfusion (Zhao *et al.*, 2003).

This form of 'stuttered' reperfusion has been demonstrated in several small clinical studies to improve myocardial reperfusion (as evidenced by ST-segment resolution, myocardial blush grade), reduce myocardial injury (as evidenced by a 40% and 47% reduction in 72 hr CK and troponin I release, respectively), reduce absolute myocardial infarct size using SPECT (by 7.7%) and improves LV ejection fraction at one year (by 7%) (Staat *et al.*, 2005; Thibault *et al.*, 2008). In this approach, following the direct deployment of a stent in the infarct-related artery, a coronary angioplasty balloon is inflated at a low pressure (4–6 kPa) for 30–60 sec and then deflated for the same length of time, a protocol which is repeated 4 times. Further larger multi-centred clinical studies are required to determine whether this invasive intervention actually improves clinical outcomes in reperfused STEMI patients.

The benefits of IPost are limited to STEMI patients receiving PCI, and so those patients reperfused by thrombolytic therapy cannot receive this form of therapy. Therefore, the administration of phar-macological agents which reproduce the cardioprotection elicited by IPost, by targeting the signal transduction pathway underlying IPost may be of potential benefit. In this regard, pre-clinical studies by our laboratory and others have identified novel targets for cardioprotection such as the Reperfusion Injury Salvage Kinase (RISK) pathway and the mitochondrial permeability transition pore (mPTP) which are amenable to pharmacological manipulation and which also underlie the cardioprotection elicited by IPost (see below).

11.3 The RISK pathway

The Reperfusion Injury Salvage Kinase (RISK) pathway refers to a group of innate pro-survival kinases, that include PI3K-Akt and MEK1/2-Erk1/2, which confer powerful cardioprotection on activation at the onset of myocardial reperfusion (Hausenloy & Yellon 2004; Hausenloy & Yellon, 2007a). Pre-clinical studies have demonstrated that the RISK pathway can be activated by a diverse number of pharmacological agents including insulin, atorvastatin, natriuretic pep-tides, erythropoietin, adipocytokines (leptin, apelin, visfatin) and so on.

The administration of any of these agents (RISK-activators) at the onset of myocardial reperfusion reduces myocardial infarct size in the region of 40–50% through the activation of the RISK pathway. Furthermore, the RISK pathway is also activated by the endogenous cardioprotective phenomena of ischaemic preconditioning and post-conditioning (Hausenloy & Yellon 2004; Hausenloy & Yellon, 2007b).

Initial proof-of-concept clinical studies have suggested that pharmacological agents such as adenosine, natriuretic peptides, erythropoietin and glucagon-like peptide 1 (GLP-1), which are known to activate the RISK pathway in pre-clinical studies, may confer cardioprotection in the clinical setting of an AMI. For example, a recent subgroup analysis of the AMISTAD II trial suggests that intravenous adenosine administered to STEMI patients receiving PCI, reduced myocardial infarct size and improved clinical outcomes in patients presenting within 3 hours of symptom onset (Kloner et al., 2006). In the J-WIND-ANP clinical study, a 3 day infusion of atrial natriuretic peptide reduced myocardial injury and improved LV systolic function in reperfused STEMI patients (Kitakaze et al., 2007). The incretin, GLP-1, has been reported to improve LV ejection fraction in STEMI patients with poor LV systolic function undergoing PCI (Nikolaidis et al., 2004). Initial safety studies suggest that high-dose erythropoietin may be capable of reducing myocardial injury in STEMI patients undergoing myocardial reperfusion. Initial clinical studies are underway examining the benefits of high–dose atorvastatin and EPO as reperfusion adjunctive therapy in STEMI patients.

However insulin, another known RISK-activator, when administered in combination with glucose and potassium as part of the GIK cocktail failed to reduce myocardial infarct size and improve clinical outcomes in a large multi-centred clinical study (Mehta et al., 2005), although a delay in the administration of the GIK therapy and a high serum glucose have been cited as potentially influencing the results (Apstein & Opie, 2005).

The mechanism through which the RISK pathway elicits its infarct-limiting effects is unclear although pre-clinical studies by our group and other have implicated the mitochondrial permeability transition pore (mPTP) as a potential end-effector (Davidson et al., 2006) (see Figure 11.1).

11.4 The mitochondrial permeability transition pore

The mitochondrial permeability transition pore (mPTP) is a critical mediator of lethal reperfusion injury, whose opening at the onset of myocardial reperfusion induces cardiomyocyte death by uncoupling oxidative phosphorylation and inducing mitochondrial swelling

(Hausenloy et al., 2003). A wealth of pre-clinical data supports this role suggesting that its opening may contribute to up to 50% of the final myocardial infarct size. Pharmacologically inhibiting its opening by administering the mPTP inhibitor, cyclosporine-A (CsA) at the onset of myocardial reperfusion has been demonstrated in animal studies to limit myocardial infarct size and prevent myocardial injury in human cardiac tissue. Furthermore, mice lacking a functional component of the mPTP sustain smaller myocardial infarcts (Lim et al., 2006). Clinical studies are now underway examining whether an intravenous bolus of CsA is capable of reducing myocardial infarct size when administered as adjunctive therapy to reperfusion in STEMI patients.

11.5 Other novel cardioprotective strategies

11.5.1 Remote ischaemic preconditioning

Inducing brief ischaemia in the arm using a blood pressure cuff has been demonstrated to reduce myocardial injury in adult patients undergoing CABG surgery, a phenomenon termed remote ischaemic preconditioning (RIPC) (Hausenloy et al., 2007) (see Chapter 7). Clinical studies are currently underway examining whether this non-invasive intervention is capable of reducing myocardial injury sustained by patients undergoing primary PCI. In particular, this intervention may be applied by paramedics in situations in which the transfer time to the cardiac centre is anticipated to be prolonged.

11.5.2 Intracoronary hyperoxaemic reperfusion

In the AMIHOT trial, patients were randomized to reperfusion with hyperoxaemic blood after primary coronary angioplasty for AMI had been successfully performed. For this purpose, arterial peripheral blood was withdrawn, mixed with aqueous oxygen and then delivered to the patient using an intracoronary infusion catheter for 90 minutes (O'Neill et al., 2007). Although no significant differences between the two study groups with regard to cardiac events and echocardiographic wall motion scores were demonstrated for the entire population, a subgroup analysis revealed smaller infarct size and greater improvement in regional wall motion for patients with anterior myocardial infarction reperfused within six hours. The AMIHOT II trial will be investigating this subgroup of patients to determine whether they benefit from this form of therapy.

11.5.3 Therapeutic cooling post-AMI

Systemic hypothermia achieved by endovascular cooling during ischaemia did not significantly reduce infarct size in two large clinical trials, although in animal experiments, myocardial cooling reproducibly results in infarct size reduction. Interestingly, in the COOL-MI study, a subgroup of patients with anterior myocardial infarction (in contrast to patients with inferior myocardial infarction), who achieved a temperature of <35°C prior to reperfusion, developed smaller infarcts (O'Neill 2003). This particular group of patients is currently been investigated in the COOL-MI II clinical study.

11.6 Conclusions

Despite current optimal therapy, the morbidity and mortality from an AMI remain significant. Promising new cardioprotective strategies such as ischaemic postconditioning and remote ischaemic preconditioning are emerging from recent small scale clinical studies. In addition, laboratory studies have identified novel cardioprotective targets which can be pharmacologically manipulated in the clinical setting to reduce myocardial injury in AMI patients. Large-scale multi-centred clinical studies are required to determine whether these new strategies for cardioprotection have the potential to improve clinical outcomes in AMI patients.

These recent developments in the research field of cardioprotection suggest that we may be at a new frontier of cardioprotection, which when considered alongside the new developments in cardiac imaging should result in continued progress in this research field.

Key references

Apstein, C.S., Opie, L.H. (2005). A challenge to the metabolic approach to myocardial ischaemia. *Eur Heart J*, **26**: 956–959.

Davidson, S.M., Hausenloy, D.J., Duchen, M.R., Yellon, D.M. (2006). Signalling via the reperfusion injury signalling kinase (RISK) pathway links closure of the mitochondrial permeability transition pore to cardio protection. *Int J Biochem Cell Biol*, **38**: 414–419.

Hausenloy, D.J., Tsang, A., Yellon, D.M. (2005). The reperfusion injury salvage kinase pathway: a common target for both ischemic preconditioning and postconditioning. *Trends Cardiovasc Med*, **15**: 69–75.

Hausenloy, D.J., Yellon, D.M. (2003). The mitochondrial permeability transition pore: its fundamental role in mediating cell death during ischaemia and reperfusion. *J Mol Cell Cardiol*, **35**: 339–341.

Hausenloy, D.J., Yellon, D.M. (2004). New directions for protecting the heart against ischaemia-reperfusion injury: targeting the Reperfusion Injury Salvage Kinase (RISK)-pathway. *Cardiovasc Res*, **61**: 448–460.

Hausenloy, D.J., Yellon, D.M. (2007a). Reperfusion injury salvage kinase signalling: taking a RISK for cardioprotection. *Heart Fail Rev*, **12**: 217–234.

Hausenloy, D.J., Yellon, D.M. (2007b). Preconditioning and postconditioning: united at reperfusion. *Pharmacol Ther*, **116**: 173–191.

Hausenloy, D.J., Mwamure, P.K., Venugopal, V., et al., (2007). Effect of remote ischaemic preconditioning on myocardial injury in patients undergoing coronary artery bypass graft surgery: a randomized controlled trial. *Lancet*, **370**: 575–579.

Kitakaze M, Asakura M, Kim J. (2007). Human atrial natriuretic peptide and nicorandil as adjuncts to reperfusion treatment for acute myocardial infarction (J-WIND): two randomized trials. *Lancet*, **370**: 1483–1493.

Kloner, R.A., Forman, M.B., Gibbons, R.J., et al., (2006). Impact of time to therapy and reperfusion modality on the efficacy of adenosine in acute myocardial infarction: the AMISTAD-2 trial. *Eur Heart J*, **27**: 2400–2405.

Lim, S.Y., Davidson, S.M., Hausenloy, D.J., Yellon, D.M. (2007). Preconditioning and postconditioning: the essential role of the mitochondrial permeability transition pore. *Cardiovasc Res*, **75**: 530–535.

Lipsic, E., van der M.P., Voors, A.A., et al., (2006). A single bolus of a long-acting erythropoietin analogue darbepoetin alfa in patients with acute myocardial infarction: a randomized feasibility and safety study. *Cardiovasc Drugs Ther*, **20**: 135–141.

Mehta, S.R., Yusuf, S., Diaz, R., et al., (2005). Effect of glucose-insulin-potassium infusion on mortality in patients with acute ST-segment elevation myocardial infarction: the CREATE-ECLA randomized controlled trial. *JAMA*, **293**: 437–446.

Nikolaidis, L.A., Mankad, S., Sokos, G.G., et al., (2004). Effects of glucagon-like peptide-1 in patients with acute myocardial infarction and left ventricular dysfunction after successful reperfusion. *Circulation*, **109**: 962–965.

O'Neill, W. Cooling as an adjunct to primary PCI for myocardial infarction. Presented at the Transcatheter Cardiovascular Therapeutics Conference, Washington, DC, September 18, 2003.

O'Neill, W., Martin, J.L., Dixon, S.R., et al., (2007). Acute myocardial infarction with hyperoxemic therapy (AMIHOT). *J Am Coll Cardiol*. **50**: 397–401.

Staat, P., Rioufol, G., Piot, C., et al., (2005). Postconditioning the human heart. *Circulation*, **112**: 2143–2148.

Thibault, H., Piot, C., Staat, P., et al., (2008). Long-term benefit of postconditioning. *Circulation* **117**: 1037–1044.

Zhao, Z.Q., Corvera, J.S., Halkos, M.E., et al., (2003). Inhibition of myocardial injury by ischemic postconditioning during reperfusion: comparison with ischemic preconditioning. *Am J Physiol Heart Circ Physiol*, **285**: H579–H588.

Index